Practical and Chemical Allergens in Contact Dermatitis

Sharon E. Jacob • Elise M. Herro

Practical Patch Testing and Chemical Allergens in Contact Dermatitis

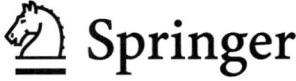

Sharon E. Jacob
Division of Dermatology
University of California
San Diego
California
USA

Elise M. Herro
Department of Dermatology
and Cutaneous Surgery
University of Texas Health
Science Center
San Antonio
Texas
USA

ISBN 978-1-4471-4584-4 ISBN 978-1-4471-4585-1 (eBook)
DOI 10.1007/978-1-4471-4585-1
Springer London Heidelberg New York Dordrecht

Library of Congress Control Number: 2012956317

© Springer-Verlag London 2013
This work is subject to copyright. All rights are reserved by the Publisher, whether the whole or part of the material is concerned, specifically the rights of translation, reprinting, reuse of illustrations, recitation, broadcasting, reproduction on microfilms or in any other physical way, and transmission or information storage and retrieval, electronic adaptation, computer software, or by similar or dissimilar methodology now known or hereafter developed. Exempted from this legal reservation are brief excerpts in connection with reviews or scholarly analysis or material supplied specifically for the purpose of being entered and executed on a computer system, for exclusive use by the purchaser of the work. Duplication of this publication or parts thereof is permitted only under the provisions of the Copyright Law of the Publisher's location, in its current version, and permission for use must always be obtained from Springer. Permissions for use may be obtained through RightsLink at the Copyright Clearance Center. Violations are liable to prosecution under the respective Copyright Law.
The use of general descriptive names, registered names, trademarks, service marks, etc. in this publication does not imply, even in the absence of a specific statement, that such names are exempt from the relevant protective laws and regulations and therefore free for general use.
While the advice and information in this book are believed to be true and accurate at the date of publication, neither the authors nor the editors nor the publisher can accept any legal responsibility for any errors or omissions that may be made. The publisher makes no warranty, express or implied, with respect to the material contained herein.

Springer is part of Springer Science+Business Media (www.springer.com)

Contents

1 Clinical Guide Introduction 1
Introduction 1
Background on Diagnostic Patch
Testing in the US 2
Allergic Contact Dermatitis (the Disease State
Once the Patient Has Developed
Contact Allergy)............................... 13
    Adolescents [Age 13–17]..................... 14
    Clinical Presentation 15
Irritant Contact Dermatitis....................... 17
Contact Urticaria 19
Protein Contact Dermatitis...................... 19
Clinical Diagnosis 20
Pre-patch Consult and Education 21
    Pediatric Patch Testing...................... 22
Procedure Outline 22
    Expected Adverse Reactions of Patch Testing... 29
Post-patch Education – Avoidance 31
Management and Therapy 31

2 Clinical Guide – Top 88 Allergens................ 35
1–2. Acrylates: Ethyl Acrylate, Methyl
Methacrylate.................................. 35
3. Bacitracin 37
4. Balsam of Peru (*Myroxylon Pereirae*) (BOP)..... 38
5. Benzalkonium Chloride 41
6. Benzophenone-3 (Oxybenzone) 42
7. Black Rubber Mix (BRM) 43

v

Contents

8–12. Caine Anesthetics (Topical): Benzocaine, Tetracaine, Dibucaine, Lidocaine, Prilocaine	45
13. Cobalt Chloride	47
14–17. Cocamidopropyl Betaine (CAPB)	51
18–19. Colophony (Rosin) and Abitol	53
20–22. *Compositae* Mix	55
23–25. Corticosteroids	57
26. Dimethyl Fumarate (DMF)	61
27–28. Disperse Dyes [Blue 106 and 124]	62
29. dl Alpha Tocopherol (Vitamin E)	63
30–31. Epoxy and Bisphenol A	64
32. Ethylenediamine Dihydrochloride (EDD)	66
33. Ethyleneurea Melamine Formaldehyde [EUMF (Fixapret Ac)]	67
34. Formaldehyde	68
35–41. Formaldehyde Releasing Preservatives (FRPs)	72
42–50. Fragrance Mix I & 51–57. Fragrance Mix II, Including 58–60. Essential Oils	74
61–63. Gallates (Propyl, Octyl, Dodecyl)	79
64. Glutaraldehyde	82
65. Gold Sodium Thiosulfate	83
66. Iodopropynyl Butylcarbamate (IPBC) or Glycacil	84
67. Lanolin (Wool wax Alcohol)	86
68. Methylchloroisothiazolone Methylisothiazolone (MCI/MI)	88
69. Methyldibromoglutaronitrile (MDBGN)	89
71. Neomycin Sulfate	90
72. Nickel Sulfate	92
73. p-Phenylenediamine (PPD)	96
74. p-Tert Butylphenol Formaldehyde Resin (PTBFR)	98
75. Paraben Mix	99
76. Potassium Dichromate	100
77. Propylene Glycol	104
78. Quinoline Mix	105

79–84. Rubber Accelerators: Carbamate,
Carba mix, Thiuram, Mercaptobenzothiazole,
Mercapto mix, Mixed Diakyl Thioureas
(Diethylthiourea and Dibutylthiourea)............ 106
85–86. Sorbitan Sesquioleate (SS)
and Sorbic Acid 111
87. Thimerosal.................................. 112
88. Tosylamide Formaldehyde Resin
or Toluenesulfonamide Formaldehyde
Resin (TSFR).................................. 114

References 115

Abbreviations

AAD	American Academy of Dermatology
ACD	Allergic Contact Dermatitis
ACDS	American Contact Dermatitis Society
AD	Atopic Dermatitis
APC	Antigen Presenting Cells
BOP	Balsam of Peru
BRM	Black Rubber Mix
CAMP	Contact Allergen Management Program
CAPB	Cocamidopropyl betaine
CARD	Contact Allergen Replacement Database
CU	Contact Urticaria
DMAPA	Dimethylaminopropylamine
DKG	German Contact Dermatitis Research Group
EDD	Ethylenediamine Dihydrochloride
EPA	Environmental Protection Agency
EU	European Union
EUMF	Ethyleneurea Melamine Formaldehyde
ICD	Irritant Contact Dermatitis
ID	Idiopathic
IPBC	Iodopropynyl butylcarbamate
IVDK	Information Network of Departments of Dermatology
MCI/MI	Methylchloroisothiazolone Methylisothiazolone
MDBGN	Methyldibromoglutaronitrile
MHC	Major Histocompatibility Complex
MSDS	Material Safety Data Sheet
NACDG	North American Contact Dermatitis Group

NIOSH	National Institute of Occupational Safety and Health
PABA	Para-aminobenzoic Acid
PCD	Protein Contact Dermatitis
PE	Phenoxyethanol
PPD	p-Phenylenediamine
PPT	Positive Patch Test
PTBFR	p-tert Butylphenol Formaldehyde Resin
PTD	Dipentamethylenethiuram Disulfide
RAST	Radioallergosorbent Test
ROAT	Repeat Open Application Test
SHMG	Sodium Hydroxymethylglycinate
SL	Sesquiterpene Lactone
SS	Sorbitan Sesquioleate
TETD	Tetraethylthiuram Disulfide
TMTD	Tetramethylthiuram Disulfide
TMTM	Tetramethylthiuram Monosulfide
TRUE Test	Thin-Layer Rapid Use Epicutaneous Test
TSFR	Toluenesulfonamide Formaldehyde Resin
UVB	Ultraviolet Light B

Chapter 1
Clinical Guide Introduction

Quote by A. Fischer [1]:

"I have indicated that in the search for causative agents of contact dermatitis the physician must literally suspect everything 'under the sun' (and the sun, itself), including those agents to which the patient has been exposed for years without prior difficulty. The patient's total environment with its flora and fauna, topical medications, clothing, cosmetics and other contactants encountered in work or play may have to be investigated. The victim must then be armed with knowledge that will enable him to distinguish friend from foe and to avoid his personal villains no matter how disguised. Thus, the victim, the patient, will be enabled to enjoy his environment with safety."

Introduction

Contact dermatitis (CD) is one of the leading reasons for patients to seek dermatology consultation, with an estimated 72 million people in the United States afflicted with this condition. There are two main types of CD, all of which result from contact of the skin or mucous membranes with an exogenous agent. The most common form of CD, accounting for ~80 % of cases, is irritant contact dermatitis (ICD), followed by allergic contact dermatitis (ACD), which represents ~20 % of cases and is the primary focus of this handbook [2–4]. Recent patch test studies in US-based populations, confirmed equal prevalence of contact allergy in pediatric and adult populations [5]. Furthermore, rates of contact allergy vary based on regional and social differences in allergen exposure, as well as differing referral patterns, selection criteria for patch testing, and allergens tested [6]. Finally, much less commonly observed are contact urticaria (CU) and protein contact dermatitis, which are beyond the scope of this handbook, but are mentioned briefly for completeness, and the reader is directed to key sources on these topics below.

Background on Diagnostic Patch Testing in the US

In the United States, Marion Baldur Sulzberger first introduced the epicutaneous patch test technique, developed by Josef Jadassohn, in the 1930's at New York Skin and Cancer Unit.

Furthermore, in 1931 Helene Ollendorff-Curth, also trained by Jadassohn, came to the United States and introduced patch testing to industries in order to improve safety measures on commercially available products. Over the next three decades, patch testing clinics were developed worldwide, and in 1962, the Scandinavian Committee for Standardization of Routine Patch Testing began to formalize patch testing procedure and materials. By the early 1980s, the Food and Drug Administration (FDA) proposed a ban on the production and sale of allergens for the patch tests based on the lack of availability of scientific evidence for its procedure, safety, and efficacy. A mandate was set for companies to standardize their medicinal chemicals.

In response, the North American Contact Dermatitis Group (NACDG) developed a research arm and worked with Stiefel Laboratories to help the German subsidiary of

Hermal receive approval for the European based Hermal/Trolab 20 standard allergen test. This test was available through the American Academy of Dermatology (AAD). Then, under the leadership of Howard Maibach and the Pharmacia-Upjohn Company, the 20 Allergen Test was transformed into what is now the commercially available Thin-layer Rapid Use Epicutaneous (T.R.U.E.) Test™ (Mekos Laboratories A/S, Hillerod, Denmark), whose first 23 allergens were approved by the FDA in 1997 [7]. By 2012, 12 new allergens/mixes had received FDA approval for commercial availability for a total of 35 chemicals/mixes.

Approximately 1,700 new synthetic chemicals on average are being brought to the U.S. market annually and, notably, the Environmental Protection Agency (EPA) tests only chemicals that demonstrate evidence of significant health risk potential. Thus, the situation is such that only about 25 % (of the 82,000 chemicals in use in the U.S.) have ever been subject to basic testing, which is why A. Fischer is astute in his observation that the physician should suspect anything and everything under the sun.

Fortunately, major culprit allergens have been identified through extensive tracking by the International Contact Dermatitis Research Group (ICDRG) and the North American Contact Dermatitis Group (NACDG) over the last 30 years. This has allowed for the compilation and generation of series of panels of allergens, which can serve as a base point to initiate screening. For example, available series include: the American Contact Dermatitis Society (ACDS) 80 Core Series [8], the fragrances series [9], the vehicle and cosmetic series [10], and then occupationally customized panels such as dentistry [11] and bakery panels [12] (see Tables 1.1, 1.2, 1.3, 1.4, and 1.5). Further series be can found on Chemotechnique Diagnostics' (Sweden) website, http://www.chemotechnique.se/Online-Catalogue.htm, or the allergEAZE™ (Calgary, AB) website, http://www.allergeaze.com/allergens.aspx?ID=Series.

As many of these allergens are found in a variety of household and cosmetic products, as well as items with which patients come in contact with daily, tailoring the patch test to patients'

TABLE 1.1 American contact dermatitis society (ACDS) 80 core series

Substance	Handbook #
1. Nickel sulfate 2.5 % pet.[a]	72
2. Myroxylon pereirae 25 % pet.[a]	4
3. Fragrance mix I 8 % pet.[a,c]	42
4. Quaternium 15.2 % pet.[a]	35
5. Neomycin 20 % pet.[a]	71
6. Budesonide 0.1 % pet.[a]	24
7. Formaldehyde 1 % aq.[a,c]	34
8. Cobalt chloride 1 % pet.[a,c]	13
9. p-tert-Butylphenol formaldehyde resin 1 % pet.[a]	74
10. P-Phenylenediamine 1 % pet.[a]	73
11. Potassium dichromate 0.25 % pet.[a,c]	76
12. Carba mix 3 % pet.[a,c]	80
13. Thiuram mix 1 % pet.[a]	81
14. Diazolidinyl urea 1 % pet.[a]	36
15. Paraben mix 12 % pet.[a]	75
16. Black rubber mix 0.6 % pet.[a]	7
17. Imidazolidinyl urea 2 % pet.[a]	38
18. Mercapto mix 1 % pet.[a]	83
19. Methylchlorisothiazolinone/Methylisothiazolinone 100 ppm. aq.[a]	68
20. Tixocortol-21- pivalate 1 % pet.[a]	23
21. Mercaptobenzothiazole 1 % pet.[a]	82
22. Colophony 20 % pet.[a]	18
23. Epoxy resin 1 % pet.[a]	30
24. Ethylenediamine 1 % pet.[a]	32
25. Wool alcohol 30 % pet.[a]	67

TABLE 1.1 (continued)

Substance	Handbook #
26. Benzocaine 5 % pet.[b]	8
27. Bacitracin 20 % pet.[a]	3
28. Mixed dialkyl thioureas 1 % pet.	84
29. Fragrance mix II 14 % pet.	51
30. Benzophenone-3.3 % pet.	6
31. Disperse blue 106.1 % pet.[a]	27
32. Disperse blue 124.1 % pet.	28
33. Gold sodium thiosulfate 0.5 % pet.[a,c]	65
34. Ethyl acrylate 0.1 % pet.	1
35. Compositae mix 6 % pet.	20
36. Sesquiterpene lactone mix 0.1 % pet.	21
37. DMDM hydantoin 1 % pet.	36
38. Tosylamide formaldehyde resin 10 % pet.	88
39. Methyl methacrylate 2 % pet.	2
40. Cinnamic aldehyde 1 % pet.	44
41. Propylene glycol 30 % aq.	77
42. Cetyl steryl alcohol 20 % pet.	N/A
43. 2-Bromo-2-nitropropane-1,3-diol (Bronopol) 0.5 % pet.[a]	39
44. Sorbitan sesquioleate 20 % pet.	85
45. Cocamidopropylbetaine 1 % aq.[c]	14
46. Glyceryl thioglycolate 1 % pet.	N/A
47. Ethyleneurea melamine-formaldehyde 5 % pet.	N/A
48. Iodopropynyl butylcarbamate 0.1 % pet.[c]	66
49. Chloroxylenol (PCMX) 1 % pet.	N/A
50. Glutaraldehyde 1 % pet.	N/A
51. Ethyl cyanoacrylate 10 % pet.	N/A

(continued)

TABLE 1.1 (continued)

Substance	Handbook #
52. Benzyl alcohol 10 %	See #4
53. Benzalkonium chloride 0.1 % aq.[c]	5
54. Methyldibromoglutaronitrile 0.5 % pet.	69
55. Propolis 10 % pet.[c]	N/A
56. n,n-Diphenylguanidine 1 % pet.	N/A
57. Lanolin alcohol (Amerchol 101) 50 % pet.	67
58. Triethanolamine 2 % pet.[c]	N/A
59. Amidoamine 0.1 % aq.	15
60. Desoximethasone 1 % pet.	See #'s 23–25
61. Triamcinolone 1 % pet.	See #'s 23–25
62. Clobetasol-17- propionate 1 % pet.	See #'s 23–25
63. Hydrocortisone-17-butyrate 1 % pet.[a]	25
64. 4-Chloro-3-cresol (PCMC) 1 % pet.	N/A
65. Benzophenone-4 2 % pet.	N/A
66. Chlorhexidine digluconate 0.5 % aq.	N/A
67. Ylang ylang 2 % pet.	N/A
68. Phenoxyethanol 1 % pet.	N/A
69. Sorbic acid 2 % pet.	N/A
70. 2, 6-Ditert-butyl-4-cresol (BHT) 2 % pet.	N/A
71. Disperse Orange 3.1 % pet.	N/A
72. 3-(Dimethylamino)propylamine (DMAPA) 1 % aq.	N/A
73. Oleamidopropyl dimethylamine 0.1 % aq.[c]	N/A
74. Dl Alpha Tocopherol 100 %	29
75. Cocamide DEA 0.5 % pet.	N/A

TABLE 1.1 (continued)

Substance	Handbook #
76. Lidocaine 15 % pet.	11
77. Dibucaine 2.5 % pet.	10
78. Jasmine absolute 2 % pet.	N/A
79. Tea tree oil 5 % pet.	N/A
80. Triclosan 2 % pet.	N/A

[a]TRUE Test allergen
[b]Caine mix (containing benzocaine) is a TRUE Test allergen
[c]Interpret reactions with caution, mild irritant and/or low clinical relevancy

TABLE 1.2 Fragrance series (perfumes/flavors)

Substance	%	Vehicle
4-(4-hydroxy-4-methyl pentyl)- 3-cyclohexene-1-carboxaldehyde (Lyral)	5	Petrolatum
Amylcinnamic alcohol	1	Petrolatum
Amylcinnamic aldeyhde	1	Petrolatum
Anisyl alcohol	1	Petrolatum
Bay leaf oil	2	Petrolatum
Benzaldehyde	5	Petrolatum
Benzyl alcohol	1	Petrolatum
Benzyl salicylate	1	Petrolatum
Benzylbenzoate	1	Petrolatum
Cinnamic alcohol	1	Petrolatum
Cinnamic aldehyde	1	Petrolatum
Citral	2	Petrolatum
Citronellal	2	Petrolatum
Citronellol	1	Petrolatum
Coumarin	5	Petrolatum

(continued)

TABLE 1.2 (continued)

Substance	%	Vehicle
d-limonene	2	Petrolatum
d-limonene	3	Petrolatum
Eugenol	1	Petrolatum
Farnesol	5	Petrolatum
Fragrance mix [A]	8	Petrolatum
Fragrance mix [B]	8	Petrolatum
Geraniol	1	Petrolatum
Hexyl cinnamic aldehyde	10	Petrolatum
Hydroxycitronellal	1	Petrolatum
Isoeugenol	1	Petrolatum
Jasminum officinale oil (jasminum grandiflorum)	2	Petrolatum
Majantol	5	Petrolatum
Oak moss absolute	1	Petrolatum
Oil cedar	10	Petrolatum
Oil neroli	2	Petrolatum
Oil of bergamot	2	Petrolatum
Oil of cinnamon	0.5	Petrolatum
Oil of cloves	2	Petrolatum
Oil of eucalyptus	2	Petrolatum
Oil of lemon	2	Petrolatum
Oil of lemon grass	2	Petrolatum
Oil of rose	0.5	Petrolatum
Oil of rosemary	0.5	Petrolatum
Orange oil	2	Petrolatum
Phenyl salicylate	1	Petrolatum
Salicylaldehyde	2	Petrolatum
Vanillin	10	Petrolatum

TABLE 1.3 Cosmetic series

Substance	%	Vehicle
1,3,5-tris(2-hydroxyethyl)-hexahydrotriazine (Grotan BK)	1	Petrolatum
2,5-diazolidinyl urea (Germall® II)	1	Petrolatum
2-bromo-2-nitropropane-1,3-diol (Bronopol)	0.5	Petrolatum
2-hydroxy-4-methoxy-benzophenone	10	Petrolatum
4-chloro-3,5-xylenol (PCMX)	1	Petrolatum
4-chloro-3-cresol (PCMC)	1	Petrolatum
Abietic acid	10	Petrolatum
Abitol	10	Petrolatum
Amerchol L101	50	Petrolatum
Benzophenone 4	10	Petrolatum
Benzyl alcohol	1	Petrolatum
Benzyl salicylate	1	Petrolatum
Butylhydroxyanisole (BHA)	2	Petrolatum
Butylhydroxytoluene (BHT)	2	Petrolatum
Cetylstearylalcohol	20	Petrolatum
Chlorhexidine digluconate	0.5	Water
Chloroacetamide	0.2	Petrolatum
Clioquinol	5	Petrolatum
Cocamidopropyl betaine	1	Water
Coconut diethanolamide (cocamide DEA)	0.5	Petrolatum
Cold cream	100	
Diethanolamine	2	Petrolatum
Dimethylaminopropylamine		Petrolatum
Diphenylthiourea	1	Petrolatum
DMDM hydantoin	1	Petrolatum
Dodecyl gallate	0.2	Petrolatum

(continued)

TABLE 1.3 (continued)

Substance	%	Vehicle
Ethylenediamine dihydrochloride	1	Petrolatum
Hexamethylenetetramine	1	Petrolatum
Imidazolidinyl urea (Germall® 115)	2	Petrolatum
Iodopropynyl butylcarbamate	0.2	Petrolatum
Isopropylmyristate	10	Petrolatum
Methylchloroisothiazinolone/methyliisothiazinolone – Kathon CG	0.01	Water
Methyldibromo glutaronitrile (MDBGN)		Petrolatum
Methyldibromo glutaronitrile/phenoxyethanol (MDBGN/PE)-Euxyl K 400	1	Petrolatum
Octyl gallate	0.2	Petrolatum
Paraben mix [B]	12	Petrolatum
Petrolatum	100	Petrolatum
Phenoxyethanol	1	Petrolatum
Phenyl salicylate	1	Petrolatum
Phenylmercuric acetate	0.05	Petrolatum
Polyethylene glycol ointment	100	
Polyethylene glycol-400	100	
Primin	0.01	Petrolatum
Propyl gallate	0.5	Petrolatum
Propylene glycol	20	Water
Quaternium 15 (Dowicil 200)	1	Petrolatum
Sesquiterpenelactone mix (2 ml)	0.1	Petrolatum
Sodium benzoate	5	Petrolatum
Sodium disulphite	1	Petrolatum
Sodium-2-pyridinethiol-1-oxide (Sodium-Omadine)	0.1	Water
Sorbic acid	2	Petrolatum

TABLE 1.3 (continued)

Substance	%	Vehicle
Sorbitan monooleate (Span 80)	5	Petrolatum
Sorbitan sesquioleate	20	Petrolatum
Stearyl alcohol	30	Petrolatum
Tea tree oil, oxidized	5	Petrolatum
Tert-butylhydroquinone	1	Petrolatum
Thimerosal	1	Petrolatum
Tolu balsam	20	Petrolatum
Tosylamide/formaldehyde resin	10	Petrolatum
Triclosan	2	Petrolatum
Trithanolaminee	2.5	Petrolatum
Tween 40	10	Petrolatum
Tween 80	10	Petrolatum
Vanillin	10	Petrolatum
Wool alcohols ointment	100	
Wool fat	30	Petrolatum

TABLE 1.4 The dentistry series (dental materials)

Substance	%	Vehicle
(2-hydroxyethyl)-methacrylate	1	Petrolatum
1,3-butandiol-dimethacrylate	2	Petrolatum
2-hydroxy-ethylacrylate	0.1	Petrolatum
2-hydroxypropyl-methacrylate	2	Petrolatum
Amalgam (Ag 13.9 %, Cu 2.4 %, Sn 3.5 %, Zn 0.02 %)	20	Petrolatum
Amalgam (Hg 2.5 %, Ag 1.7 %, Cu 0.3 %, Sn 0.4 %, Zn 0.025 %)	5	Petrolatum
Ammoniated mercury	1	Petrolatum
Ammonium tetrachloroplatinate	0.25	Petrolatum

(continued)

TABLE 1.4 (continued)

Substance	%	Vehicle
Benzoyl peroxide	1	Petrolatum
BIS-GMA	2	Petrolatum
Bisphenol A	1	Petrolatum
Bisphenol-A-dimethacrylate	2	Petrolatum
Copper sulphate	1	Water
Diurethane-dimethacrylate	2	Petrolatum
Ethyleneglycol-dimethacrylate	2	Petrolatum
Eugenol	1	Petrolatum
Mentha piperita oil (peppermint oil)	2	Petrolatum
Methyl methacrylate	2	Petrolatum
N,N-dimethyl-p-toluidine	2	Petrolatum
Palladium chloride	1	Petrolatum
Potassium dicyanoaurate	0.002	Petrolatum
Sodium thiosulfoaurate (gold)	0.25	Petrolatum
Tetracaine-HCl	1	Petrolatum
Tin (II) chloride	0.5	Petrolatum
Triethyleneglycol-dimethacrylate	2	Petrolatum

TABLE 1.5 The bakery series

Substance	Conc. %	Vehicle	Conc. molality (m)
Vanillin	10.0	Petrolatum	0.657
Eugenol	2.0	Petrolatum	0.122
Isoeugenol	2.0	Petrolatum	0.122
Sodium benzoate	5.0	Petrolatum	0.347
BHT	2.0	Petrolatum	0.091
Menthol	2.0	Petrolatum	0.128

TABLE 1.5 (continued)

Substance	Conc. %	Vehicle	Conc. molality (m)
Cinnamyl alcohol	2.0	Petrolatum	0.149
Cinnamal	1.0	Petrolatum	0.151
2-tert-Butyl-4-methoxyphenol (BHA)	2.0	Petrolatum	0.111
Trans-Anethole	5.0	Petrolatum	0.337
Sorbic acid	2.0	Petrolatum	0.178
Benzoic acid	5.0	Petrolatum	0.409
Propionic acid	3.0	Petrolatum	0.405
Octyl gallate	0.25	Petrolatum	0.009
Dipentene (oxidized)	1.0	Petrolatum	0.073
Ammonium persulfate	2.5	Petrolatum	0.110
Benzoylperoxide	1.0	Petrolatum	0.041
Propyl gallate	1.0	Petrolatum	0.047
Dodecyl gallate	0.25	Petrolatum	0.007

specific exposure history can be very effective when used in conjunction with an appropriately broad-based screening panel. Customizing patch testing chambers allows for a comprehensive approach to testing by placing specific allergens or product samples into individual chambers on separate panels then applying the panels to unaffected regions of the patient's back.

Allergic Contact Dermatitis (the Disease State Once the Patient Has Developed Contact Allergy)

ACD is a complex immunologic reaction that ultimately results in a delayed (~48–120 h) presentation, referred to as a Type IV hypersensitivity reaction. This immune response is characterized by two main stages, sensitization and elicitation. An individual may become sensitized to a particular substance when his or her skin barrier is impaired, allowing for the entry of exogenous allergens into the epidermis. These allergens or haptens are small, lipophilic chemicals with low molecular weight (<10,000 Da) that bind with self proteins to form complete antigens upon entry into the epidermis. Dendritic cells, which are the antigen presenting cells (APCs) of the skin, then uptake and express these complete antigens on cell surface major histocompatibility complexes (MHC). The antigen is then presented by dendritic cells to naïve antigen-specific T-cells in the regional lymph nodes. These naïve T-cells then differentiate into effector/memory T-cells, which are capable of acting on APC's in the future [13–16].

Elicitation, the second phase of ACD, refers to the clinical dermatitic presentation, and occurs after repeated exposure to a particular allergen to which memory T-cells have been cloned. Exposure may occur transepidermally or systemically through ingestion, inhalation or intravenous entry [17]. In this stage, T-helper cells dominate as opposed to T-suppressor cells, which would create a state of relative or complete tolerance [16].

Because this process is delayed, patients may have difficulty discovering or temporally associating the initial source of their dermatitis, especially if it was years prior; therefore, patch test screening with an appropriate base panel is of utmost importance. Moreover, the distribution of the dermatitis may not follow the exposure pattern. ACD can present as a local, generalized, or ectopic dermatitis.

Adolescents [Age 13–17]

Childhood presentations of ACD are becoming more recognized as a significant problem, accounting for approximately 20 % of all cases of pediatric dermatitis [15, 16]. Moreover, adolescents account for a large proportion of pediatric ACD, especially in females when compared to their male counterparts, according to international literature. This trend has been observed with particular allergens, such as nickel and fragrance,

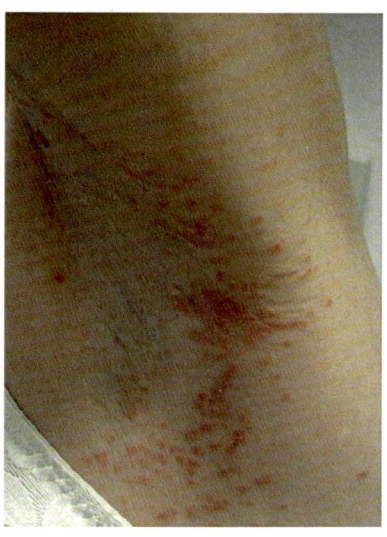

FIGURE 1.1 Sparing of axillary vault with allergic contact dermatitis

likely due to their presence in classically female sources, i.e. jewelry, cosmetics, and fragranced personal products [16, 18]. Recent studies, however, have reported an even distribution of allergens across all pediatric groups without noting gender bias [19, 20]. One relevant source of ACD in adolescents is sports equipment, i.e. wrist supports, shin and knee guards [21–23], athletic tape [24], and swimming goggles [25], often due to the allergen p-tert-butylphenol formaldehyde resin [26]. In addition, the warm, moist, occluded environment to which athlete's skin is subjected, may also make them more susceptible to ACD. The moisture may also contribute to chemical breakdown and release of allergens [27].

Clinical Presentation

ACD often presents with pruritic, eczematous papules and plaques, and occasional vesicles and bulla (Figs. 1.1, 1.2, 1.3, and 1.4). Because these descriptive terms are not unique to ACD, distinguishing it from AD and ICD can prove to be a challenge [16]. More specifically, acute ACD and AD often have similar morphological appearances, and furthermore,

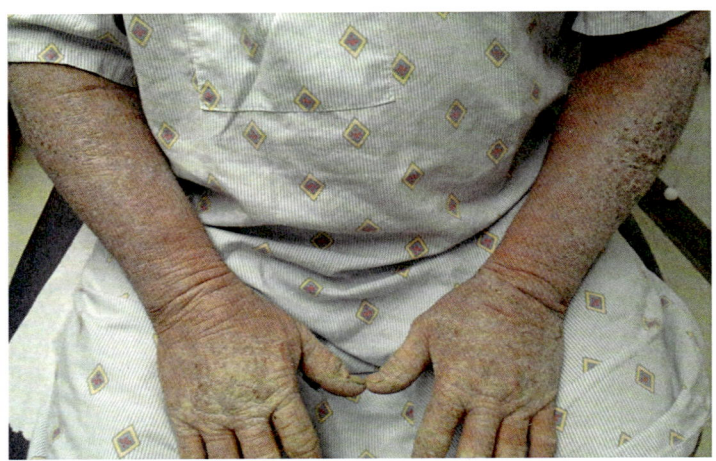

Figure 1.2 Erythroderma from advanced allergic contact dermatitis

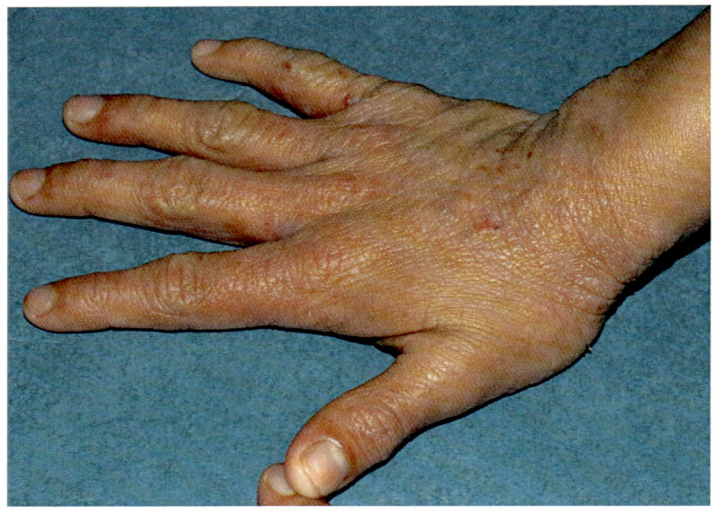

Figure 1.3 Allergic contact hand dermatitis

the two may occur simultaneously. In fact, it has been suggested that AD may predispose individuals to developing ACD due to a damaged epidermal barrier to allergens [28, 29]. Acute presentations of ACD and ICD may be distin-

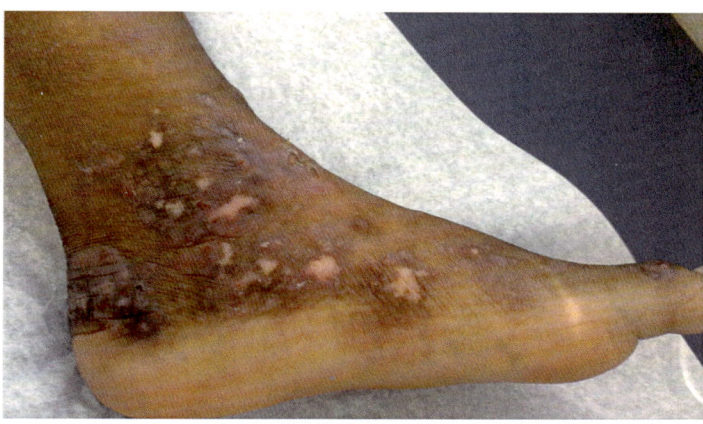

FIGURE 1.4 Chronic, allergic contact dermatitis of the foot, with lichenification and scarring

guished based on their temporal relationship to the inciting event as well as clinical distribution (see Table 1.6) [15, 16, 30]. ACD may present in an ectopic manner, meaning that the location of the dermatitis is not directly related to exposure site. This can occur in different ways, such as by transferring an allergen from one region of the body to another. For example, AD sites may flare after exposure to nail polish upon scratching [29] or eyelid dermatitis may ensue after a cashier rubs his or her eyes after handling monies. Even more challenging to diagnose are idiopathic (id) ACD reactions, which are non-specific, widespread eruptions that occur when the patient contacts a particular allergen [15, 16].

Irritant Contact Dermatitis

ICD is not considered an immunologic reaction, but rather is related to direct contact with an irritating substance that damages epidermal keratinocytes and induces inflammation, without activating an immune cascade. Therefore, previous chemical exposure and prior sensitization are not required for this reaction [31]. Classic examples of irritants include urine (diaper dermatitis), soap (hand dermatitis), and saliva

TABLE 1.6 Differences between acute ACD vs. acute ICD

Type of dermatitis	Temporal relationship to the inciting event	Clinical distribution	Symptoms
Allergic contact	Delayed hypersensitivity reaction	Induration or papulovesicular eruptions often expand beyond the location of contact	Usually pruritus
	Often presenting 48 h to up to 3 weeks	Ectopic patterns can be observed	
		Idiopathic (id) reactions are possible	
Irritant contact	Usually within 24 h	Appears as well-demarcated, erythematous, and sometimes follicular papules and plaques	Usually burning
	Concentration of the offending substance is inversely related to time of onset	Usually confined to areas of contact exposure	

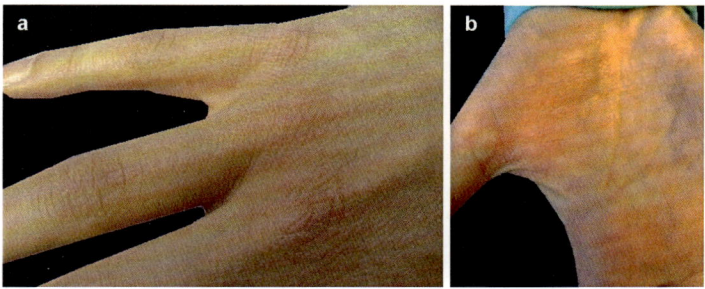

FIGURE 1.5 Irritant contact dermatitis of the dorsal (**a**) and palmar (**b**) surfaces of the hand

(lip licker dermatitis) (Fig. 1.5). Moreover, the severity of an ICD reaction is not solely dependent on the concentration of the instigating agent, but is directly proportional to the exposure time as well [15, 32].

Contact Urticaria

Unlike the type IV delayed immunologic reaction of ACD, CU is mediated by an immediate IgE type I immunologic reaction. Clinically, CU appears as a wheal and flare reaction, appearing within 30 min of exposure to a eliciting substance and resolving within hours [33]. Testing is usually performed by an allergist, who uses the RAST (radioallergosorbent test) or prick testing. Desensitization can then be attempted, which is much more difficult with Type IV reactions [16].

Protein Contact Dermatitis

The term protein contact dermatitis (PCD) was introduced in 1976 by Hjorth and Roed-Peterson [34], and refers to the development of a Type-I, immediate, IgE-mediated reaction upon exposure to protein. Clinically, the most common presentation of PCD is chronic or recurrent eczema; however, urticaria may also be observed upon contact with particular proteins, such as certain foods and drinks (almonds, banana, carrot, celery, kiwi, melon, tomato, seafood, cow's milk), airborne ragweed particles, and natural rubber latex [33, 35].

Clinical Diagnosis

Investigative history and diagnostic clues are important elements to making a proper diagnosis of ACD. For instance, distinguishing between ACD and AD can be challenging, especially when occurring simultaneously. Luckily, certain clinical clues can increase the index of suspicion for ACD, such as new-onset, and/or a progressing or deteriorating dermatitis that is recalcitrant to standard therapies [36]. Epicutaneous patch testing, however, is the gold standard for the diagnosis of ACD [15, 16, 30] (see Table 1.7) [15, 28].

TABLE 1.7 Allergen determination for comprehensive patch testing

Patient history	Clinical pattern of dermatitis

Personal hygiene products
  Patient
  Close contacts (due to connubial dermatitis)
	Local: dermatitis may relate to region of direct contact, i.e. peri-umbilical dermatitis linked to nickel allergy due to jean snaps and belts

Home environment	Ectopic: dermatitis may relate to region of indirect contact, i.e. peri-ocular dermatitis after rubbing eyes with nail polish
Medical history	Skin memory: dermatitis presents in region of previous exposure upon re-exposure to source at a different site, i.e. ingestion of chocolate (containing nickel) causes a peri-umbilical reaction
	Systemic, generalized: widespread appearance of dermatitis after systemic exposure, i.e. ingestion, intravenous, intramuscular, inhalation

Pre-patch Consult and Education

In the pre-patch education/instruction session, a provider must explain basic guidelines prior to testing (see Table 1.8) [36] as well as the testing procedure. As these instructions can be extensive, patients may not be willing or able to follow these rules. Therefore, a basic explanation of ACD being a delayed reaction in the initial consultation often helps patients to understand the lengthy testing timeline. There may be some patients, however, that do not appear capable of understanding all of the instructions and explanations, and the provider must then assess whether they would be a proper candidate as well [28]. Not only may the test itself be inaccurate based on patient's inability to follow instruction, but subsequent attempts at avoidance may not be possible.

TABLE 1.8 Patch testing guidelines

Guideline	Timeline
No creams or lotions on their back or pre-determined application site	Day of testing through final interpretation
No showering (cannot get application sites wet)	Application to final interpretation
No excessive sweating	Application to final interpretation
No topical steroids or topical calcineurin inhibitors on predetermined application site	1–2 weeks prior to application through final interpretation
No oral corticosteroids	Within 2 weeks prior to patch testing and through final interpretation
No IM corticosteroids	Within 4 weeks prior to patch testing and through final interpretation
No sun or UV light on the area to be tested	Weeks prior to testing through final interpretation
Oral antihistamines are allowed	Prior to and during testing

Pediatric Patch Testing

Pediatric patch testing poses more of a challenge when compared to testing adult patients. Selectivity of proper candidates not only includes taking a patient's age into account, but their family's ability to understand the process and their willingness to complete the journey. In addition, patch testing itself can be limited by the relatively smaller surface area available for chamber application (especially in dermatitic patients). Therefore, there is an increased need for selectivity when choosing which allergens to include in the series. Logistically, it is also difficult to ask a young child to sit still for a long period of time during patch application, removal, and interpretation. Moreover, patients' parents or legal guardians must be made aware that the procedure has not received Food and Drug Administration indication in pediatric patients [28]. Preliminary avoidance of allergens with a high likelihood of reactivity is especially helpful with pediatric patients, as testing may not be necessary if the patient has shown >50 % improvement in their condition in 4–6 weeks of avoidance. This also allows for a snapshot of the family's ability to comply with an avoidance plan.

Procedure Outline (see Fig. 1.6)

Patch testing can be achieved by using either commercially available pre-packaged allergen panels or by loading each allergen onto individual chambers on a tape strip. Some types of the patient's own products may also be applied directly to patch testing chambers, and placed on patients in addition to individual component chemicals [37] (Fig. 1.7). Panels of allergens and/or products should be placed on unaffected areas of patient's backs or arms in linear configurations and marked according to a pre-determined number scheme (Figs. 1.8 and 1.9). Securing these panels with hypoallergenic tape, such as hypafix tape ™ (Smith & Nephew, London, UK), is crucial, as these strips of allergens must remain in place under occlusion for 24–48 h. The 48 h point was selected to allow for optimized time of contact with the substance without increasing the

- **Step 1:** Place pre-packaged or pre-loaded allergen panels on unaffected areas of patient's back or anterior arms.

- **Step 2:** Mark each allergen with a surgical marker according to a pre-determined number scheme

- **Step 3:** Create a paper "map" of panel configuration and numbering

- **Step 4:** Secure panels with hypoallergenic tape

- **Step 5:** Remove panels between 24–48 hours, outlining each allergens' position with a fluorescent marker and re-numbering with a surgical marker

- **Step 6:** Note early reactions and their intensity, macular erythema, 1+, 2+, 3+ (See **Table 1–9**)

- **Step 7:** Perform final interpretation at 72–120 h from initial placement, noting consistent or new reactions according to the same scale as before, using a wood's lamp to illuminate the fluorescent marking

Figure 1.6 Patch testing algorithm

number of irritant reactions [38]. Of note, the German Contact Dermatitis Research Group (DKG) suggests a 24 h contact time for children ages 6–12.

An initial reading of the patch testing sites is performed upon removal of the allergen panels at the 48 h point and outlining individual chambers with a fluorescent marker (Fig. 1.10). Skin changes, such as erythema, induration, papules, vesicles, and blistering are noted at this time, and

24 Chapter 1. Clinical Guide Introduction

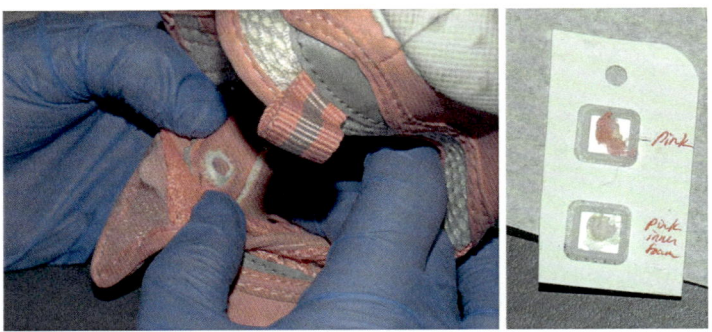

FIGURE 1.7 Sample from an athletic shoe is removed using a punch biopsy instrument, dissected into parts, such as cloth and foam, and placed in patch testing chambers

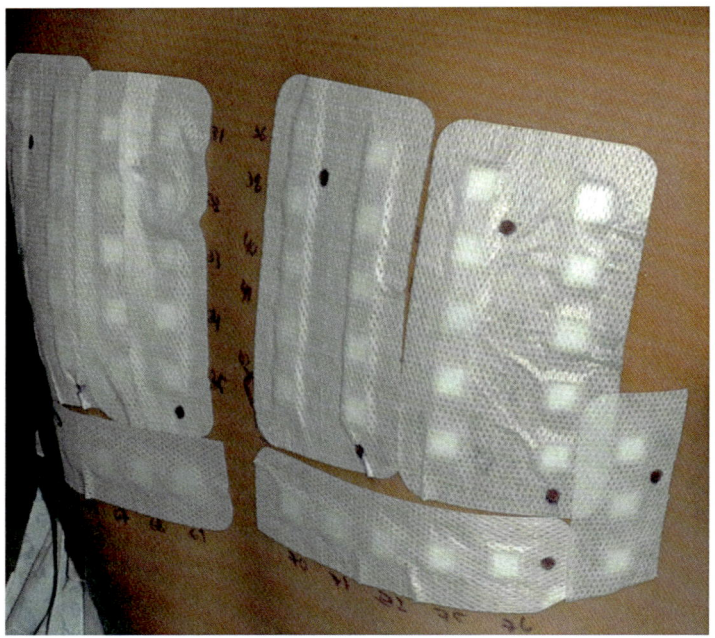

FIGURE 1.8 Patch test application. Panels of allergens placed in linear configurations and marked according to a pre-determined number scheme

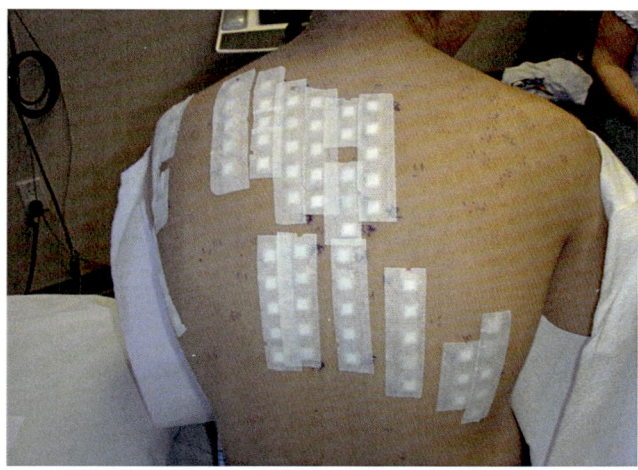

FIGURE 1.9 Avoidance of marked regions due to pre-existing dermatitis

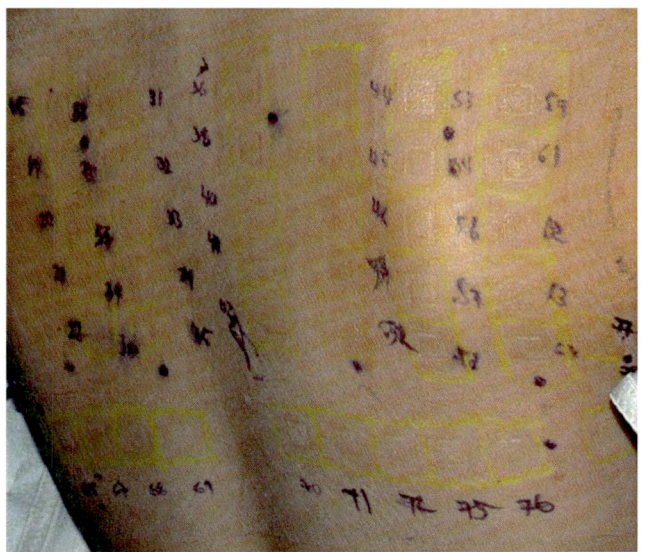

FIGURE 1.10 Patch test removal. An initial reading of the patch testing sites is performed at the 48 h point, with chambers outlined in highlighter and each allergen re-numbered with surgical marker

TABLE 1.9 Reaction rating scale

Macular erythema	Faint to pronounced erythema without elevation
1+	Induration +/− erythema
2+	Papules +/− induration and erythema
3+	Vesicles and/or bulla +/− papules, induration and erythema

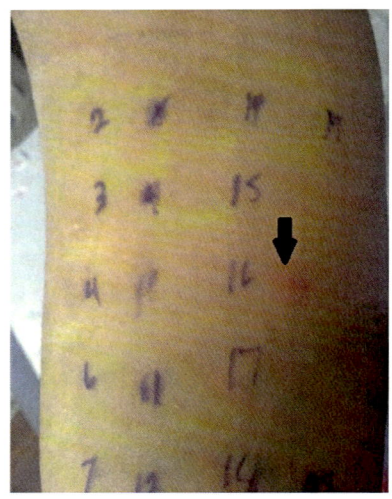

FIGURE 1.11 Final interpretation, macular erythematous reaction (*arrow*) to p-tert butylphenol formaldehyde resin (PTBFR)

rated accordingly. Reactions may range in intensity from macular erythema to a 3+ positive patch test (PPT) (see Table 1.9). However, the final interpretation must be done at a delayed reading in 72–120 h from initial placement, as initial cutaneous changes may be due to ICD, of which the majority resolve by the final interpretation (Figs. 1.11, 1.12, 1.13, and 1.14). In addition, 48 h may not be long enough for some of these type IV delayed reactions to appear or peak in intensity [15, 16]. Notably, corticosteroids, neomycin sulfate, and sodium gold thiosulfate appear late (see Table 1.10) [39, 40]. The final interpretation can be aided by the use of a wood's lamp, which will illuminate the highlighter in order to locate and directly feel the patch testing sites (Fig. 1.15).

Procedure Outline 27

FIGURE 1.12 Final interpretation, 2+ reaction to bacitracin (*arrow*)

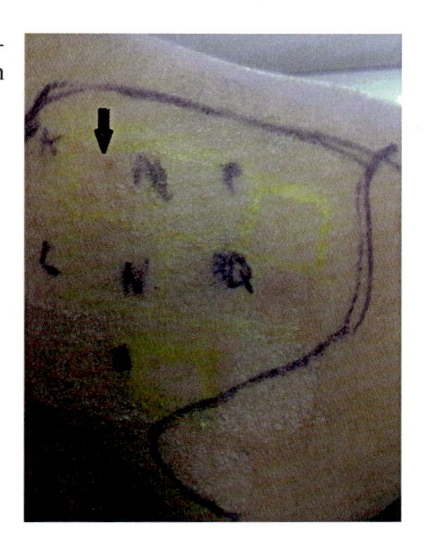

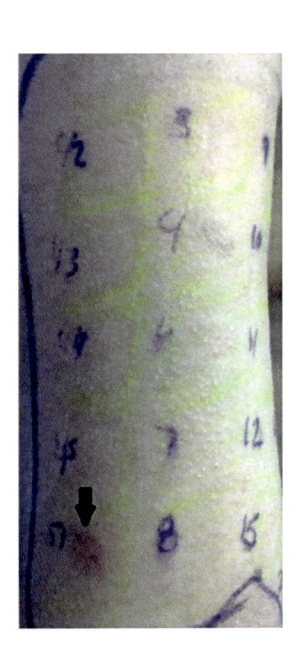

FIGURE 1.13 Final interpretation, 2+ reaction cobalt chloride

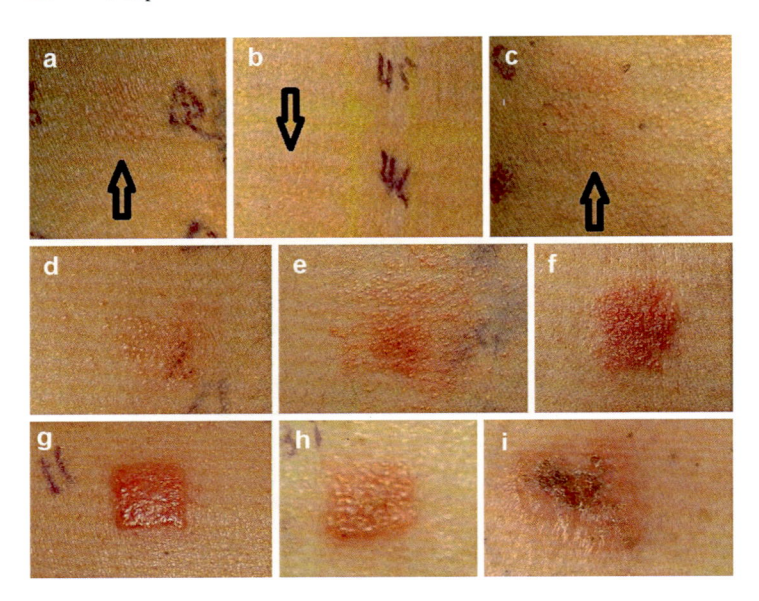

FIGURE 1.14 Reactions. (**a**) macular erythema; (**b**) macular erythema; (**c**) 1+ reaction; (**d**) 1+ reaction; (**e**) 2+ reaction; (**f**) 2+ reaction; (**g**) 2+ reaction; (**h**) 2+ reaction; (**i**) 3+ reaction

TABLE 1.10 Early vs. late reactions

Early reactions	Late reactions	Crescendo reactions
Balsam of Peru (*Myroxylon pereirae*)	Acrylates	Cocamidopropyl betaine
Carbamates	Compositae	
Thiuram	Corticosteroids (budesonide)	
	Formaldehyde releasing preservatives	
	Neomycin sulfate	
	Sodium gold thiosulfate	
	Textile dyes	

FIGURE 1.15 Final interpretation with the use of a wood's lamp to illuminate the highlighter in order to directly feel the patch testing sites

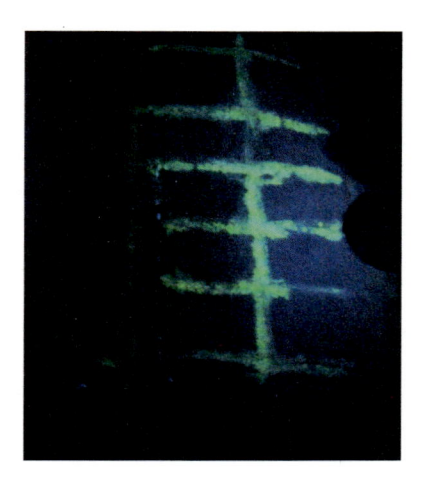

Certain chemicals and products, however, are not designed to be used under occlusion or to remain in contact with a patient's skin for long periods of time, and for that reason, a provider may decide to test particular products by employing provocative use testing. This form of testing, also called, repeat open application testing (R.O.A.T.) utilizes the inner or anterior arm of the patient, and involves placing a small amount of the product in question to a 2.5 cm drawn circle twice daily for 7 days (see Fig. 1.16). Importantly, this technique does not involve occluding chemicals as in classic patch testing; therefore, the allergen potency is not as great, which decreases risk of intense reactions, but also may require longer time to elicit a response.

Expected Adverse Reactions of Patch Testing

The most common adverse reactions associated with patch testing are expected cutaneous changes at the sites that were in contact with the testing substances, especially if the patient exhibited contact allergy (PPT). These reactions may include erythema, induration, papules, and vesicles, occasionally accompanied by pruritus, burning and inflammation at the site of application.

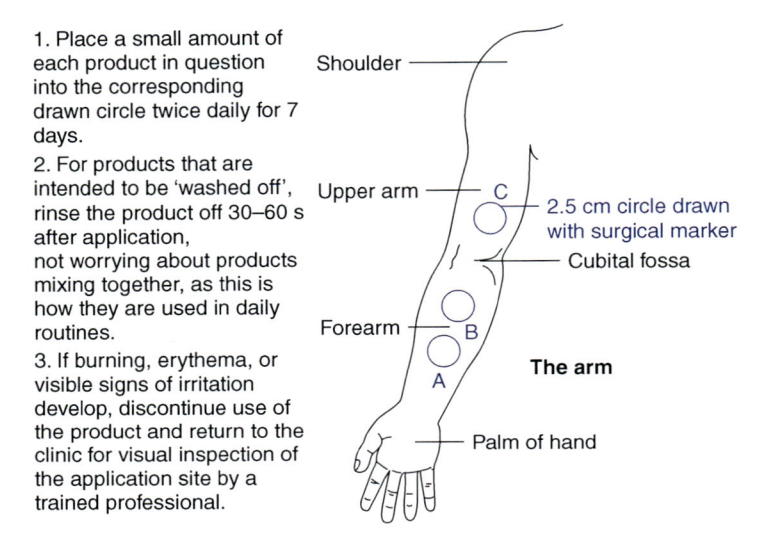

1. Place a small amount of each product in question into the corresponding drawn circle twice daily for 7 days.
2. For products that are intended to be 'washed off', rinse the product off 30–60 s after application, not worrying about products mixing together, as this is how they are used in daily routines.
3. If burning, erythema, or visible signs of irritation develop, discontinue use of the product and return to the clinic for visual inspection of the application site by a trained professional.

FIGURE 1.16 Repeat open application testing (R.O.A.T.)

Less commonly seen are pustular and blistering reactions, post-inflammatory hypo/hyper-pigmentation, and persistent granulomatous reactions. The most rare of reactions would be anaphylactic type reactions, which have been reported as individual case reports in which the patients have had contact urticarial syndrome (Type I) or developed a Type I hypersensitivity reaction to the agent. Some patients may experience a worsening of their initial dermatitis, which can serve as a diagnostic clue in assigning clinical relevance, as this phenomenon can be observed when one is tested and reacts to the same allergen that contributed to the initial and current presentation.

Moreover, based on information extrapolated from adult studies, active sensitization to one of the allergens tested at the standardized concentrations are very rarely reported (0.0–0.69 %) [40–43]. Published concentrations of chemicals used in commercially available patch testing kits are associated with the fewest side effects and are generally accepted [44]. Ultimately, the potential risks and side-effects presented by patch testing are considerably outweighed by its usefulness, both as a diagnostic tool and as a guide to avoiding clinically relevant specific contact allergens.

Post-patch Education – Avoidance

While patch testing can provide a diagnosis of ACD and facilitate discovery of culprit allergens, it is patients that are responsible for the resolution of their dermatitis. This is because ***avoidance*** is crucial in the treatment of ACD, and can only be achieved with proper patient education. A post-patch testing session is necessary to inform the patient and their families of potential sources of exposure based on a thorough explanation of what their clinically relevant, positive allergens are and where they are often found. Patient-directed literature is available and should be provided to patients to aid in this endeavor. As there are endless products commercially available, teaching patients how to read the ingredient labels is also important, but there are online databases available for this purpose as well. Individualized lists of "safer" alternatives can then be generated, by entering relevant, positive allergens into the database [28]. Both programs also offer information about various allergens. There are two main programs that can provide this service, the Contact Allergen Management Program (C.A.M.P.) and the Contact Allergen Replacement Database (C.A.R.D.) [45, 46]. Products on these listings should be used with caution, however, as patients are generally not patch tested for every chemical ingredient. For this reason, educating the patient and family on performing provocative use testing or R.O.A.T. should be performed.

Management and Therapy (see Fig. 1.17)

Avoidance of causative allergens is the most crucial component of ACD resolution and management [47]. As mentioned earlier, patch testing can provide a means of discovering

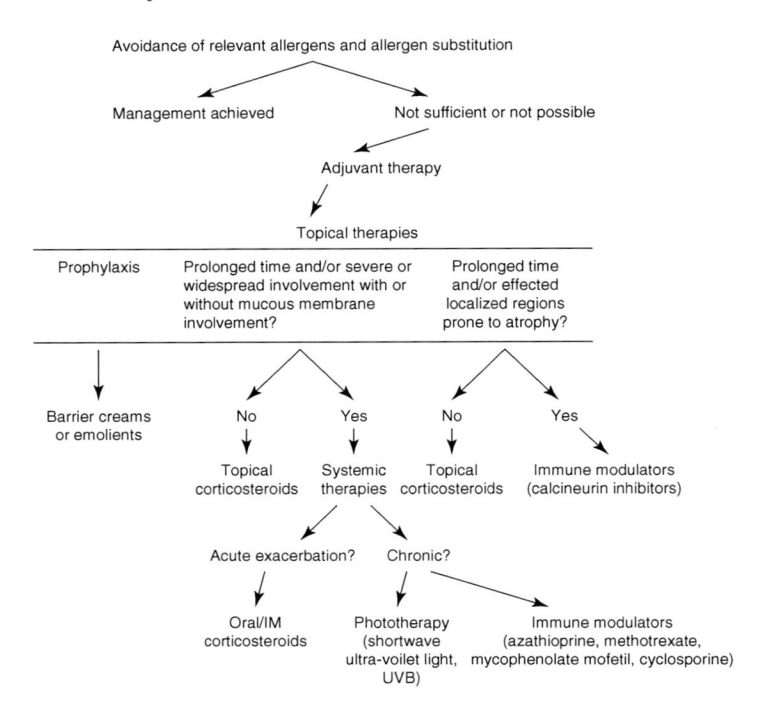

```
                    Avoidance of relevant allergens and allergen substitution
                   ←───────────────────────────────────────────────→
       Management achieved                              Not sufficient or not possible
                                                            ↓
                                                     Adjuvant therapy
                                                            ↓
                                                     Topical therapies
───────────────────────────────────────────────────────────────────────────────
Prophylaxis    Prolonged time and/or severe or        Prolonged time
               widespread involvement with or         and/or effected
               without mucous membrane                localized regions
               involvement?                           prone to atrophy?
───────────────────────────────────────────────────────────────────────────────
    ↓              ↙         ↘                          ↙         ↘
Barrier creams    No          Yes                      No          Yes
or emolients      ↓            ↓                        ↓           ↘
              Topical      Systemic                 Topical     Immune modulators
              corticosteroids  therapies            corticosteroids  (calcineurin inhibitors)
                           ↙        ↘
                  Acute exacerbation?  Chronic?
                          ↓              ↓
                      Oral/IM         Phototherapy      Immune modulators
                      corticosteroids (shortwave       (azathioprine, methotrexate,
                                      ultra-voilet light,  mycophenolate mofetil, cyclosporine)
                                      UVB)
```

FIGURE 1.17 Management algorithm

relevant, positive allergens, allowing a provider to focus post-patch education on how to avoid specific chemicals [28, 47]. Patients are also educated on allergen substitution, which is aided by certain resources, such as the Alternatives for the 2007 NACDG Standard Screening Tray [48] and a 4-part series providing data from the American Contact Alternatives Group [49–52]. This series focuses on facial cosmetics, hair products, lip and dental care products, as well as personal care products. With these interventions, it may be possible to achieve a sustained remission.

There are times, however, when complete avoidance is not possible or when avoidance is not sufficient to clear a dermatitis outbreak. Moreover, patch testing may fail to identify any or all inciting agents, especially if multiple chemicals are involved. Adjuvant measures, such as topical and/or systemic therapies may be necessary in these instances. In addition, physical barrier creams or emollients, such as petrolatum, can be utilized in many different situations as a form of exposure avoidance or prophylaxis. Topical agents are used as first line therapy, specifically corticosteroids, which may elicit side effects or induce sensitization to the vehicle ingredients or corticosteroids themselves with prolonged or widespread use [53–55]. Due to the issues surrounding long-term use of topical corticosteroids, topical immune modulators, such as calcineurin inhibitors [56, 57], may prove beneficial, especially in regions of thin skin or those prone to atrophy, such as the face and intertriginous areas. The next step in management involves the use of systemic therapies, which may be necessary for severe or widespread dermatitis with or without mucous membranes manifestations, or for dermatitis that continues to progress despite the use of topical agents.

Oral corticosteroids, such as prednisone [58], can be effective for acute exacerbations of ACD and tapered after symptoms are controlled. For chronic cases, however, 'steroid sparing' agents should be considered, such as phototherapy, usually with shortwave ultra-violet light (UVB), and systemic immune modulators (azathioprine, methotrexate, mycophenolate mofetil, and cyclosporine) [47].

Chapter 2
Clinical Guide – Top 88 Allergens

1–2. Acrylates: Ethyl Acrylate, Methyl Methacrylate

Description: chemicals naturally found in liquid or powder form that harden into solid substances when heat is applied or additional chemicals are added. ACD to acrylates is caused by the free acrylate monomer, which is reduced once the resin has hardened [59].

Sources: often occupational exposures [60, 61]

Acrylic nails
Aircraft windows
Bone cement – orthopedics
Concrete
Dental products

- Cements
- Crowns, temporary
- Dentures

Gel electrophoresis
Glass
Hair spray
Industrial adhesives/glues
Inks, ultraviolet-cured
Insecticides

Paints, ultraviolet-cured
Plastics
Textile finish

Allergen of the Year: N/A

Degree of Relevance: high (~80 %), but low prevalence; the NACDG reported the prevalence of PPTs to ethyl acrylate and methyl methacrylate as 1.3 % and 1.4 % of their patients, respectively [62]. Acrylates can penetrate most latex, nitrile, neoprene, and vinyl gloves within minutes, so protection can be difficult. Therefore, polyvinyl alcohol and barrier chemical resistant gloves should be used.

Classic Presentation: related to site of exposure, especially in liquid or powder form.

Potential Ectopic Dermatitis: Yes, due to acrylic fingernails in contact with eyelids, mouth, neck, and genitalia.

Potential Generalized/Systemic Dermatitis: N/A

Co-reactivity/Cross-reactivity: Possible cross-reactions among some acrylates.

Test:

Patch test

3. Bacitracin

Description: topical antibiotic that is now site #33 on the T.R.U.E. Test.
 Sources:

Animal feeds
Over-the-counter medications – ointments and creams

Allergen of the Year: 2003
Degree of Relevance: high
Classic Presentation: site of application, i.e. eczema sites, wounds
Potential Ectopic Dermatitis: unlikely
Potential Generalized/Systemic Dermatitis: rare; however, it can cause anaphylaxis [63]
Co-reactivity/Cross-reactivity: co-reactivity with neomycin (see #71)
Test:

Patch test
Repeat Open Application Test (ROAT)

4. Balsam of Peru (*Myroxylon Pereirae*) (BOP) (Table 2.1)

Description: fragrance/flavorant found in nature from the sap of the *Myroxylon pereirae* tree, containing >400 chemicals, and one of the chemicals used to screen for fragrance allergy [36, 65]. BOP can be found at site #10 on the T.R.U.E. Test.

As mentioned above, allergy to fragrance was first published in the medical literature in 1957 [66] and flavorants in 1961 [67]. Since that time, multiple reports have been documented.

TABLE 2.1 Components of balsam of Peru (partial list) [64]

a-amylcinnamic alcohol[a]

Cinnamic alcohol[a]

Cinnamic aldehyde[a]

Eugenol[a]

Isoeugenol[a]

Benzaldehyde

Benzoic acid

Benzoyl benzoate

Benzoyl cinnamte

Benzoyl salicylate

Benzyl alcohol

Cinnamic acid

Methyl cinnamate

Sodium benzoate

Vanillin

[a]Component of fragrance mix I as well

4. Balsam of Peru (Myroxylon Pereirae) (BOP)

Sources [68, 69]:

Cosmetics
Creams
Dental Items – mouthwash, dental floss, toothpaste
Diaper-area care products
Foods and drinks containing Balsam of Peru (*Myroxylon pereirae*) (Table 2.2) [18, 70, 71]
Lotions
Lozenges
Medications (flavored liquid)
Perfumes

TABLE 2.2 Foods and drinks containing balsam of Peru (*Myroxylon pereirae*)

Desserts	**Drinks**	**Fruits and vegetables**	**Spices**
Chocolate	Alcohol	Citrus fruit products	Allspice
	Beer	Baked goods	
	Gin	Jams	
	Vermouth	Juices	
	Wine		
Ice cream (vanilla extract)	Soda (flavorants and preservatives)	Tomato and tomato products: barbeque sauce, chili, ketchup, tomato sauce	Anise
			Cinnamon
			Cloves
			Curry
			Ginger
			Vanilla

Allergen of the Year: N/A
Degree of Relevance: high (children and adults)
Classic Presentation: ACD on the face (eyelids), neck and axillae, as well possible stomatitis or cheilitis [72, 73] are common presentations. BOP also may be associated with hand dermatitis [74], and diaper dermatitis, as children may become sensitized through the use of baby products used in the diaper region or the diaper's components themselves [75, 76].

Oral and perioral dermatitis are often caused by the BOP flavorings in chewing gums, toothpastes, mouthwashes, and mentholated cigarettes [75]. In addition, as components of BOP are used in fragrances as well, "consort" or "connubial" contact dermatitis also can occur by contact with others, such as partners, care-givers, friends or co-workers, who use fragranced products [77].

Potential Ectopic Dermatitis: Potentially
Potential Generalized/Systemic Dermatitis: Yes; Airborne contact, and dermatitis due to systemic exposure by inhalation and ingestion (flavor and spices in foods) may also occur [70, 74, 77, 78].
Co-reactivity/Cross-reactivity: cross-reactivity fragrance mix I and II and colophony (see #'s 42, 51, and 18)
Test:

Patch test – while many products, such as cosmetics and creams, may be tested "as is," products such as dental and flavored items, may require preparation prior to patch testing [79].
Repeat Open Application Test (ROAT)

5. Benzalkonium Chloride

Description: quaternary ammonium cationic detergent used as both a preservative and antiseptic [80].

Sources:

Antiseptic solutions and detergents, i.e. Zephiran
Cosmetics
Deodorants
Dentrifices – mouthwashes
Lozenges
Medicated towelettes and adhesive tapes
Ophthalmic solutions – contact lens solutions and eye drops
Orthopedics – Plaster of Paris (antiseptic component), rare [80, 81]

Allergen of the Year: N/A

Degree of Relevance: low

Classic Presentation: related to site of contact, including stomatitis

Potential Ectopic Dermatitis: unlikely

Potential Generalized/Systemic Dermatitis: Yes, when sensitized individuals ingest antihypertensive or antispasmodic medications that cross-react benzalkonium chloride [80].

Co-reactivity/Cross-reactivity: cross-reactivity with some antihypertensive or antispasmodic medications

Test:

Patch test
Repeat Open Application Test (ROAT)

6. Benzophenone-3 (Oxybenzone)

Description: the most common photoallergen in sunscreen products, causing ACD or contact urticaria. Several benzophenones exist with a variety of uses, such as protection from ultraviolet light [82].

Sources:

Sunscreen/sunblock

Allergen of the Year: N/A
Degree of Relevance: high
Classic Presentation: related to the site of contact.
Potential Ectopic Dermatitis: N/A
Potential Generalized/Systemic Dermatitis: unlikely
Co-reactivity/Cross-reactivity: Cross-reactivity with ketoprofen possible [83].

Test:

Patch test
Repeat Open Application Test (ROAT)

7. Black Rubber Mix (BRM)

Description: BRM contains the three antioxidants, N-isopropyl-N'-phenyl paraphenylenediamine, N-cyclohexyl-N'-phenyl paraphenylenediamine, and N,N'-diphenyl paraphenylenediamine, which are added to rubber in order to produce the black pigment. These chemicals are oxidized themselves in order to prevent damage to the rubber molecules [84]. They also provide temperature stability, strength, and flexibility [84].

As early as 1943, ACD to rubber accelerants was reported by E.E. Obetz, who coined the term "rubber itch" or "rubber poisoning" [85]. BRM now occupies #16 on the T.R.U.E. Test panel, and the NACDG reported that 38 % of those with PPT's to a rubber mix were reactive to BRM [86]. Moreover, sensitization to BRM in the general population is approximately 2.1 % in men and 1.6 % in women [86]. The use of vinyl gloves may add protection to those sensitized to BRM.

Rubber is derived from the sap of the tree, *Hevea brasiliensis*, sometimes referred to as the "rubber tree." This sap is also used in natural latex, and while ACD to rubber additives (accelerators, antidegradants, antioxidants, fillers, reinforcing agents, retarders, and vulcanizers) is common, so too are type I immediate reactions to the latex protein [86, 87].

Sources: [88] many black rubber products, but the black pigment is not necessarily present in products containing BRM [86]

    Car steering wheel
    Condoms
    Earphones
    Erasers
    Factory conveyor belts
    Industrial rubber

- Tires
- Automotive belts

    Makeup sponges
    Medical equipment: gloves, stethoscopes

Paints
Pest repellants
Playgrounds – recycled tire shreddings were used as fillers in the 1990's prior to reports of sensitization and the subsequent replacement of this substance [89, 90]
Rubber bands, boots, handles and escalator handrails [91], indwelling catheters (can be replaced with silicone)
Shoes
Sports equipment – goggles, handles, snorkel masks, balls
Underwear elastic and rubberized waistbands (especially when washed with bleach)
Watch bands
Wheelchair padding
Wire insulation

Allergen of the Year: N/A
Degree of Relevance: moderate
Classic Presentation: related to site of contact
Potential Ectopic Dermatitis: unlikely

Potential Generalized/Systemic Dermatitis: Yes; these chemicals may become aerosolized during heating and pressurizing [86]

Co-reactivity/Cross-reactivity: PPD (see #73), as well as the rubber accelerators, carbamate, mercaptobenzothiazole, mercapto mix, and thiruam, as these chemicals are often used together [86]. Moreover, patients with contact allergy to disperse textile dyes (see #'s 27 and 28) may show concomitant PPTs to BRM and PPD [92]. These dyes are derivatives of PABA, much like PPD, whose derivatives are present in BRM.

Test:

Patch test – may be accomplished with the actual sample of rubber as well, as long as the product is intended for prolonged use on skin, such as the watch strap.

8–12. Caine Anesthetics (Topical): Benzocaine, Tetracaine, Dibucaine, Lidocaine, Prilocaine

Description: local anesthetics composed of either *esters* (benzocaine, tetracaine) or *amides* (lidocaine, prilocaine, dibucaine). The ester anesthetics are derived from para-aminobenzoic acid (PABA). Patch testing for caine allergies can be accomplished using a "caine mix," which contains 2 esters and 1 amide, i.e. benzocaine, tetracaine hydrochloride, dibucaine hydrochloride, respectively [93]. This mix is located on site #5 on the T.R.U.E. Test.

Sources:

Topical anesthetics used to alleviate/help a wide variety of conditions:
Arthritis – creams/gels
Foot conditions – athlete's foot (tinea pedis), calluses, corns
Oral conditions – cold sores, denture irritation, teething pains, toothaches, lip balms, sore throats (cough drops, lozenges and sprays)
Skin – cuts, dermatitis (Poison Ivy), hemorrhoids, insect bites, pruritus (anti-itch creams), sunburns

Allergen of the Year: N/A

Degree of Relevance: Ester anesthetics cause ACD relatively frequently compared to amide anesthetics [93]; however, the vehicle used to deliver the anesthetic could be responsible to the reaction as well, such as parabens in lidocaine [94].

Classic Presentation: related to the site of contact with the allergen.

Potential Ectopic Dermatitis: unlikely

Potential Generalized/Systemic Dermatitis: rare, reported with benzocaine [95].

Co-reactivity/Cross-reactivity: Cross-reactivity between ester anesthetics is common; whereas, cross-reactivity between amide anesthetics and between esters and amides in uncommon [96]. Therefore, if a patient is found to have a contact allergy to an ester, an amide anesthetic can generally be substituted if necessary. Moreover, due to the low cross-reactivity between amide anesthetics, if a patient is found to be allergic to a particular amide anesthetic, a different amide may be utilized [93]. Cross-reactivity between the PABA derivatives, *ester* anesthetics, and other PABA-like derivatives found in sunscreens and creams, PPD based permanent hair dyes (see #73), aniline dyes, hydrochlorothiazide, sulfonamide antibiotics, as well as sulfonylurea diabetic medications [97, 98].

Test:

Patch test
Repeat Open Application Test (ROAT)

13. Cobalt Chloride

Description: ubiquitous, brittle, hard, white metal, often used as an alloy with nickel [99], and can increase overall strength. Cobalt, however, is not an abundant metal in nature, but traces or more are mined with many other metals, such as nickel, iron, copper, lead, and silver. Cobalt is often used to impart a blue color to objects. This chemical is included in the T.R.U.E. Test at site #12.

Sources [100]:

Brass
Cements
Ceramics
Coal
Copper
Clothing – snaps, buttons, zippers
Dental amalgams and equipment
Dyes
Fertilizers
Foods containing cobalt [101, 102] (Table 2.3)
Gold alloys (particularly white gold)
Greases (heavy duty)
Jewelry, costume (earrings, necklaces, etc.)
Joint replacements
Kitchen utensils
Makeup pigments
Medical equipment
Metal-plated objects
Nickel
Oils – mechanic and machinist
Orthodontic braces
Paints/Pigments (cobalt blue)
Potters clay
Scissors
Soil
Tattoo pigments (blue) (Fig. 2.1)
Varnishes
Vitamins (B12/*cyanocobalamine)*

TABLE 2.3 Foods containing cobalt

Animal products	Seafood	Fruits and nuts	Vegetables and beans	Grains	Drinks and desserts
Kidney[a]	Clams[a]	Apricots	Beets	Barley	Beer
Liver[a]	Ocean fish	Figs[a]	Cabbage	Buckwheat[a]	Cocoa and chocolate[a]
Meats[a]	Oysters[a]	Nuts, especially Brazil[a]	Legumes (peas and beans, especially garbanzo beans and chickpeas)[a]	Oats	Coffee
Milk[a]	Scallops		Lettuce	Seeds[a]	Soy milk[a]
	Sea vegetables		Spinach	Whole-grain flour	Tea

[a]Richest sources of cobalt

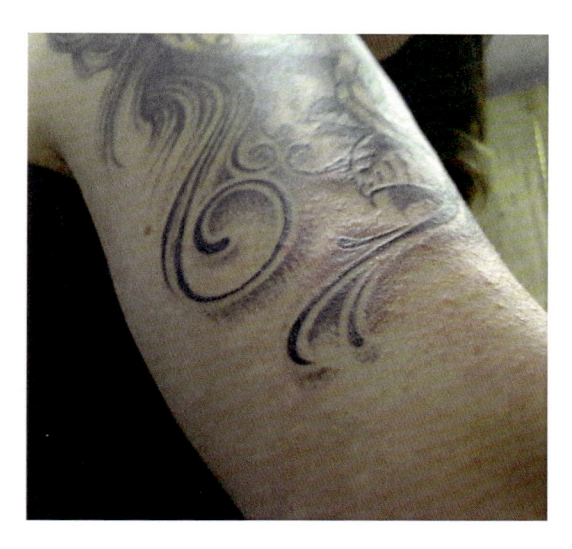

FIGURE 2.1 Allergic contact dermatitis to the blue ink (cobalt) in this patient's tattoo

Allergen of the Year: N/A
Degree of Relevance: high
Classic Presentation: similar to nickel, i.e. earlobes, neckline, umbilical area, and hands, as well as oral manifestations.
Potential Ectopic Dermatitis: Yes
Potential Generalized/Systemic Dermatitis: Yes, systemic exposure through oral intake of cobalt has caused dermatitis flares [74, 102]
Co-reactivity/Cross-reactivity: Co-reactivity with nickel (see #72) and potassium dichromate (see # 76)
Test:

Patch test; Punctate purpura can be seen in response to cobalt chloride (Fig. 2.2)
Confirmatory cobalt detection testing kit, containing disodium-1-nitroso-2-naphthol-3,6-disulfonate able to identify cobalt release at 8.3 ppm [103–105]

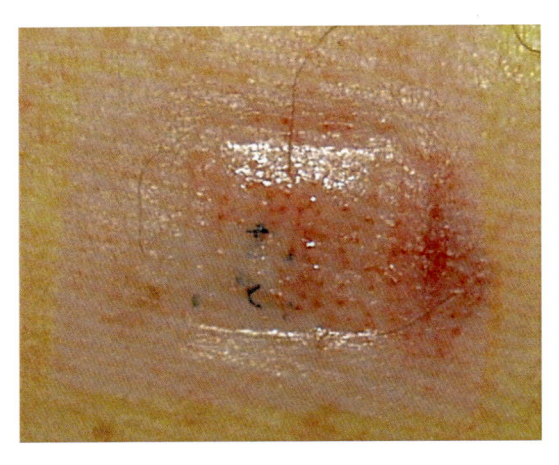

FIGURE 2.2 Punctate purpura in response to cobalt chloride

14–17. Cocamidopropyl Betaine (CAPB)

Description: a surfactant derived from coconut oil that is an emerging contact allergen, especially among those with atopic dermatitis [106]. Supplemental patch testing with manufacturing intermediates, **15. amidoamine** (cocamidopropyl dimethylamine) and **16. dimethylaminopropylamine (DMAPA)**, can be useful, as these impurities may be responsible for sensitization [107, 108]. Moreover, DMAPA can also be found in amindoamine, as well as in other fatty acid amidoamines, such as **17. oleamidopropyl dimethylamine**. In addition, as surfactants may act as irritants, delayed reading of patch test results is crucial.

Sources [36, 109]:

Bath gel/foam
Cleansers (foaming)
Contact lens solutions
Detergents (liquid, laundry)
Make-up removers
Shampoos ('no tear' formulations), including pet shampoos
Soaps (liquid)
Toothpaste

Allergen of the Year: 2004
Degree of Relevance: high
Classic Presentation: Head, neck, and facial region, but it can also be associated with other sites of contact (Fig. 2.3).
Potential Ectopic Dermatitis: unlikely
Potential Generalized/Systemic Dermatitis: Yes
Co-reactivity/Cross-reactivity: Cross-reactivity with the manufacturing contaminants, *amidoamine* [110, 111] and *3-dimethylaminopropylamine* (DMAPA) [112, 113], which are byproducts that can be the true sensitizers in CAPB. Due to this concern, cosmetic manufacturers are being encouraged to remove these impurities [114].
Test:

Patch test
Repeat Open Application Test (ROAT)

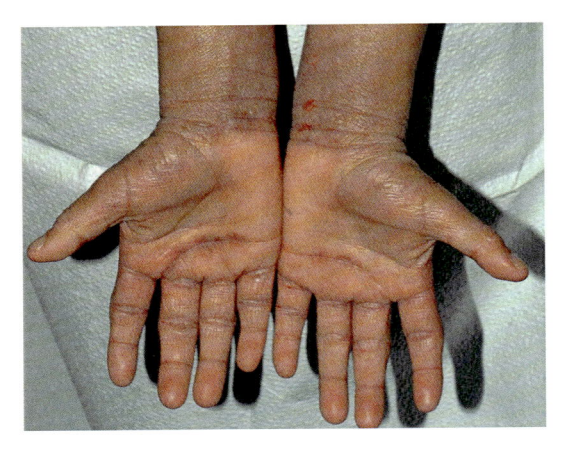

FIGURE 2.3 Anterior wrist and palmar allergic contact dermatitis to cocamidopropyl betaine (CAPB) and bronopol

18–19. Colophony (Rosin) and Abitol

Description: a sticky, amber resin from the distillation products of pine and spruce trees, composed of mostly *pimaric acid* and *abietic acid* [115]. Occupational ACD is largely observed in jewelers, machine operators, carpenters, electricians, instrumental musicians, and dentists. It is located in the #7 position of the T.R.U.E. Test.

Sources [115]:

Adhesives, adhesive plasters, glues, -ostomy appliances, postage stamps, and tapes
Asphalt products
Cements (linoleum, rubber, shoe, thermoplastic tile)
Chewing gum
Cleaners for leather and office machines
Corrosion inhibitors (automobile cooling systems, brake-shoe lining)
Cosmetics – mascaras, lipsticks, eyeshadows, concealer, eyebrow wax
Cutting oils
Dentistry: Rosin in chloroform solution is used as varnish for pulp protection in deep cavities. It also has been added to zinc oxide or eugenol in pulp capping preparation surgical packs and impression pastes. In addition, rosin is used in dental and periodontal dressings, dental cement, and liquids and cavity varnish as well as dental floss.
Diapers (top layer)
Fillers (putty, wood dough)
Fireworks
Grease remover for clothes
Ink – pens, printing
Match tips
Modeling clay
Nail polish
Paints
Paper – coating on paper, glossy paper, photographic paper, price labels, plastics and stickers. Rosin can increase water

resistance and prevent feathering or spreading of ink.
Personal hygiene products – creams, hair pomade, soaps (brown, yellow, and transparent)
Pine extracts
Polish (floor, furniture, metal, shoe, car)
Polythene (polyethylene) Sawdust and pine tree resin
Sealants
Shoes
Solvents
Stains
Tacky/powdered substances – to prevent slipping. This applies to the automobile industry, belts on machinery, rosin bag for baseball players, handles for sports, string coating of musical instruments (violin), dancer's shoe tips, floors of studios and stages.
Varnishes
Waterproofing agents
Wax – sealing, shoe, grafting, car, floor, furniture, hair removal

Allergen of the Year: N/A
Degree of Relevance: moderate
Classic Presentation: directly related to site of contact
Potential Ectopic Dermatitis: unlikely
Potential Generalized/Systemic Dermatitis: Yes

Co-reactivity/Cross-reactivity: Co-reactivity with fragrance mix I & II, balsam of Peru (both cross-reactivity as well) [116]. Components of colophony and balsam of Peru naturally occur together, such as in tomatos, which contain coniferyl alcohol (colophony) and cinnamic alcohol (balsam of Peru), and both may be incorporated into fragrances [18, 20]. Cross-reactivity may also be seen with **19. abitol**, as it produced from abietic acid [117].

Test:

Patch test

20–22. *Compositae* Mix

Description: *Compositae* is plant Family, also referred to as the *Asteraceae* Family, with >20,000 different species of flowers, herbs, vegetables and weeds [118], representing 10 % of the world's flowering plants. Seasonal dermatitis is common with allergy to this family, worsening in the summer. **Sesquiterpene lactones (SLs)** and **parthenolide** are extracts from these plants (Table 2.4).

The allergenicity of the *Compositae* Family largely comes from its essential oils, sesquiterpenes, of which the lactone subtype is most responsible for ACD. Parthenolide, a component of *Parthenium* genus (feverfew), is an example of a SL [118]. It has been shown to inhibit platelet aggregation and the release of serotonin from platelets, events that can be associated with migraines [119].

One testing or screening substance for contact allergy to *Compositae/Asteraceae* is **sesquiterpene lactone mix**, which contains three lactones; however, this mix alone is not sufficient to detect all sensitized individuals [120]. For this reason, **20. *Compositae* mix** and **21. sesquiterpene lactone mix** can be used together as screening substances. **22. Parthenolide**, now site #34 on the T.R.U.E. Test, is also an option to screen for allergy to this plant Family, but does not significantly alter the detection rate when used as a supplement to SL mix [121].

Sources:

Cosmetics
Food/drinks – teas (chamomile, sunflower, chrysanthemum) [122]
Herbal supplements

Allergen of the Year: N/A
Degree of Relevance: moderate
Classic Presentation: corresponds to exposure pattern, such as airborne contact
Potential Ectopic Dermatitis: N/A
Potential Generalized/Systemic Dermatitis: Yes, through oral intake, e.g. tea [123], or inhalational exposure due to the airborne nature of some of these plant allergens [124]

TABLE 2.4 Members of the *Compositae* family (Common names)

Arnica

Artichoke

Burdock

Chamomile (including German)

Chicory

Chrysanthemum

Daisy

Dandelion

Feverfew

Lettuce

Marigold

Ragweed

Sunflower

Co-reactivity/Cross-reactivity: There is a high rate of cross-sensitization among the SL's due to similar chemical structures; therefore, patch testing to specific members of the family can be a challenge due to false positive results [125, 126].

Test:

Patch test
Repeat Open Application Test (ROAT)

23–25. Corticosteroids

Description: encompasses five groups of corticosteroids, separated based on structure, with differing sensitization potentials [A (5.72 %)>B (4.80 %)>D1 (3.54 %)>D2 (2.13 %)>C (1.10 %)] [127–131] (see Table 2.5). Class A corticosteroids include over-the-counter products, i.e. Cortaid, Cortizone-10, as well as the patch testing screening substance, **23. tixocortol-21-pivalate**, which is #27 on the T.R.U.E. Test. The higher prevalence of sensitization to this class is likely due to its increased accessibility. **24. Budesonide** (site #30 on the T.R.U.E. Test) and triamcinolone are the screening substances for class B, and **25. hydrocortisone-17-butyrate** (T.R.U.E. test site #31) for class D2.

More recently, a new molecular grouping of corticosteroids was suggested, which only includes three groups and reflects previous cross-reactivity between classes (see Table 2.6) [132].

Sources:

Medication – oral, inhaled/nasal spray, topical spray, cream, ointment, drops (optic/otic)

Allergen of the Year: 2005

Degree of Relevance: High (0.2–6 % of patients have been found to display ACD to one of five groups of corticosteroids [133–136]); Contact allergy to corticosteroids is now more recognized in children [137, 138].

Classic Presentation: low corresponds to body site of contact.

Potential Ectopic Dermatitis:

Potential Generalized/Systemic Dermatitis: Yes, systemic corticosteroids can suppress a reaction caused by topical corticosteroids at doses >20 mg in an adult. Notably, in patients allergic to the corticosteroids they relate resolution of dermatitis at higher doses (suppressive effect of the steroid) and flaring upon weaning down the dose.

Co-reactivity/Cross-reactivity: Potential co-reactivity with sorbitan sesquioleate (see #85). Cross-reactions between group A and D2, as well as between certain corticosteroids in group B and group D2 are possible [136, 139, 140].

Test:

Patch test
Repeat Open Application Test (ROAT)

TABLE 2.5 Structural classes

Structural class[a]	Members	Patch test substance	Possible cross-reactors
Class A: Hydrocortisone type	Cortisone, fludrocortisone, hydrocortisone, hydrocortisone acetate, methylprednisolone acetate, prednisolone, prednisone, tixocortol-21-pivalate	Tixocortol-21-pivalate	Class D2
Class B: Triamcinolone acetonide type	Amcinonide, budesonide, desonide, flucinonide, fluocinolone acetonide, triamcinolone acetonide, halcinonide, triamcinolone diacetate	Budesonide, triamcinolone acetonide	Budesonide cross-reacts with D2
Class C: Betamethasone type	Betamethasone, clocortolone, desoximetasone, dexamethasone, dexamethasone sodium phosphate		

Class D1: Betamethasone dipropionate type	Alcometasone dipropionate, betamethasone dipropionate, betamethasone valerate, clobetasol-17-propionate, clobetasone butyrate, diflorasone diacetate, fluticasone propionate, hydrocortisone-17-valerate, mometasone furoate	Clobetasol-17-propionate
Class D2: Methylprednisolone aceponate type	Hydrocortisone-17-butyrate, hydrocortisone buteprate, hydrocortisone valerate, methyl-prednisolone aceponate, prednicarbate	Hydrocortisone-17-butyrate
		Class A and budesonide

[a]Grouped based on structure, not potency

TABLE 2.6 Molecular groups

Group	1	2	3
Molecular modeling & cross-reactivity grouping	The non-methylated, most often non-halogenated molecules (Formerly Group A, D2 and budesonide)	The halogenated molecules with a C16/C17 cis ketal/diol structure (Formerly acetonide Group B)	The halogenated and C16-methylated molecules (Formerly Group C and D1) that only rarely produce allergy
Testing substance	Tixocortol-21-pivalate	Triamcinolone acetonide	Desoximethasone
	Hydrocortisone 17-butyrate		Clobetasol-17-propionate
	Budesonide		

26. Dimethyl Fumarate (DMF)

Description: the methyl ester form of fumaric acid and an extremely potent irritant and sensitizer [141, 142] used in desiccant and anti-mold sachets/pouches [143, 144]. In addition, a mixture of fumaric acid esters has been used as an oral treatment of psoriasis [142].

Sources [145]:

Furniture (sachets) – sofas, chairs
Shoes [146, 147] – sachets in boxes and shoe constituents [142]
Textiles – jeans, hats [142]

Allergen of the Year: 2011

Degree of Relevance: moderate; In March 2009, the European Commission banned the importation of products contaminated with DMF; the maximum allowed amount of DMF in a given item was set at 0.1 mg/kg (0.1 ppm) [148].

Classic Presentation: related to sites in contact with furniture or shoes, i.e. posterior body (backs and buttocks), face (laying on couches), and feet

Potential Ectopic Dermatitis: unlikely

Potential Generalized/Systemic Dermatitis: After oral intake, epigastralgia, vomiting, nausea, and diarrhea have been noted, as well as a flushed face, headache, fatigue, a feeling of warmth, and lymphopenia.

Co-reactivity/Cross-reactivity: Cross-reactivity to acrylates and methacrylates [141] (see #2)

Test:

Patch test

27–28. Disperse Dyes [Blue 106 and 124]

Description: aniline dyes with sensitizing potential [149], as they are partially water soluble and easily leached out of fabrics onto the skin with normal wear and repeated washing [106, 150]. For this reason, they are often used to screen for textile dermatitis in adult and pediatric patients. The T.R.U.E Test now includes disperse blue 106 at site #35.

Sources [151]:

Clothing – including undergarments, primarily used to color polyester, acetate and nylon fibers
Diapers [152]
Eyeglass frames [153]
Seatbelts [154]

Allergen of the Year: 2000
Degree of Relevance: moderate to high
Classic Presentation: related to body location in contact with item, often peri-axillary bands and diaper edge
Potential Ectopic Dermatitis: unlikely
Potential Generalized/Systemic Dermatitis: unlikely
Co-reactivity/Cross-reactivity: Cross-reactivity to p-Phenylenediamine (see #73)
Test:

Patch test: with individual dyes, as well as with a swatch of the patient's suspect garment directly applied to the skin, as many colors can make up a hue

29. dl Alpha Tocopherol (Vitamin E)

Description: natural substances that are prone to oxidation, but are still sometimes used as pure antioxidants in foodstuffs. Most vegetable oils and animal fats contain tocopherols in their natural state. It is the topical application of Vitamin E that causes ACD or contact urticaria rather than ingestion.
Sources:

Creams
Deodorant

Allergen of the Year: N/A
Degree of Relevance: low
Classic Presentation: related to the site of exposure.
Potential Ectopic Dermatitis: potential transfer if agent is in a cream preparation
Potential Generalized/Systemic Dermatitis: no reports
Co-reactivity/Cross-reactivity: N/A
Test:

Patch test
Repeat Open Application Test (ROAT)

30–31. Epoxy and Bisphenol A

Description: a resin first manufactured and introduced in the 1930's, often used as an adhesive and surface protectant [155]. Epoxy resin is located at site #14 on the T.R.U.E Test. It can penetrate rubber gloves, so heavy vinyl gloves are recommended for protection or use of epoxy-free bonding agents.

There are different types of epoxy resins, such as uncured epoxy resins, an example being the sensitizer **31. Bisphenol A** (acetone-phenol condensation). It is the uncured epoxy resin that presents an allergy risk, as opposed to the cured epoxy resin. Cured epoxy resins, however, require addition of hardeners, such as amine hardener, which are potent sensitizers. Therefore, amide or anhydride hardeners are preferred. Epoxy resins may also be blended with urea-formaldehyde, phenol-formaldehyde, and melamineformaldehyde to form additional sensitizing agents.

Sources [155, 156]:

Adhesives and glues, all purpose (metal cements, model making)
Aircrafts
Automotive primers
Canned food tin coating
Ceramics
Dental bonding agents
Electrical – encapsulation/insulation for transformers, coils, and motors
Electronics – cell phones, game boys, laptops, iPods
Fiberglass (addition of epoxy to glass fibers) – boats, cars, suspension bridges
Finishes (appliances, roads, bridges) and varnishes
Flame retardants
Floorings (laminate)
Formica (composite of epoxy and quartz) – furnishings
Medical equipment (hemodialysis, pacemakers)
Paints
Pipe and tank linings

Polyvinyl chloride films (stabilizers and plasticizers); beads in necklaces; handbags; Plastic/vinyl gloves; Plastic panties
Sculpting
Tapes
Wall panel coatings

Allergen of the Year: N/A

Degree of Relevance: moderate, but allergy rates are low, since most consumer products contain cured epoxy resins, decreasing sensitivity. Of more concern, are raw epoxy materials, such as epichlorohydrin and bisphenol-A, used in many factories, posing an occupational exposure.

Classic Presentation: Related to site of contact

Potential Ectopic Dermatitis: unlikely

Potential Generalized/Systemic Dermatitis: Breathing epoxy fumes should be avoided, so as to prevent potential systemic exposure.

Co-reactivity/Cross-reactivity: Bisphenol-A may cross-react with diethylstilbestrol and silicone products. Amine hardeners may cross-react with ethylenediamine hydrochloride (EDD) (see # 32)

Test:

Patch test

32. Ethylenediamine Dihydrochloride (EDD)

Description: EDD, also referred to as 1,2-Ethanediamine Dihydrochloride and 1,2-Diaminoethane Dihydrochloride Chlorethamine, is a stabilizer and precursor chemical to some antihistamines, such as piperzine [157, 158].

Sources:

Cleaners (engine, toilet bowl)
Creams (anti-fungal, corticosteroid combinations, as well as antihistamine creams)
Fungicides, herbicides, and insecticides
Industrial – corrosion retardants, lubricants, solvents, and resin adhesive
Medications – aminophylline (asthma), ophthalmic solutions and nasal spray containing antihistamine
Rubber accelerators (stabilizers)

Allergen of the Year: N/A
Degree of Relevance: moderate (included in T.R.U.E. Test #11)
Classic Presentation: related to site of exposure
Potential Ectopic Dermatitis: unlikely

Potential Generalized/Systemic Dermatitis: Yes, upon exposure to cross-reacting antihistamines, patients may develop dermatitis.

Co-reactivity/Cross-reactivity: Cross-reactivity to some first-aid products, as well as antihistamines and anti-nausea medications, such as the piperazines (hydroxyzine) and cetirizine, as well as promethazine and meclizine, respectively. Zinc pyrithione in anti-dandruff shampoos may also cross-react.

Importantly, the following medications are free of EDD: anti-asthma (theophylline), antihistamine (diphenhydramine, fexofenadine, loratadine), and topical creams (doxepin, nystatin/triamcinolone acetonide (Mycolog II)) [157].

Test:

Patch test
Repeat Open Application Test (ROAT)

33. Ethyleneurea Melamine Formaldehyde [EUMF (Fixapret Ac)]

Description: a relatively newer textile resin, when compared to urea formaldehyde resin (UF), melanine formaldehyde (MF), and ethylene urea (EU). As of 2008, dimethylol dihydroxyethylene urea [DMDHEU (Fixapret CPN)] was described as the best or recommended screening test for the US market [48, 159, 160]. Although, Fowler et al. has also recommended EUMF for use as a textile dermatitis screening tool [161].

Sources:

Textiles – clothing, uniforms, upholstery

Allergen of the Year: N/A

Degree of Relevance: moderate

Classic Presentation: Related to region of contact, especially areas of the body that may rub against clothing, i.e. posterior neck, axillae and body folds [162].

Potential Ectopic Dermatitis: unlikely.

Potential Generalized/Systemic Dermatitis: unlikely if the allergic reaction is only to the resin itself and not the free formaldehyde component.

Co-reactivity/Cross-reactivity: This depends on whether the patient reacts to the formaldehyde or the EUMF itself [162, 163].

Test:

Patch test

34. Formaldehyde

Description: preservative with antimicrobial properties, used in the cosmetic industry with an average concentration between 0.02–0.03 % [164]. It is listed by the U.S. Environmental Protection Agency (EPA) as a "probable carcinogen," [165] and is prohibited in Sweden and Japan for use in cosmetics. It is an irritant as well as a top contact allergen for both adults and children, with increasing rates of sensitization [19, 166]. Studies have demonstrated that levels of free formaldehyde as low as 200–300 ppm (0.02–0.03 %) in cosmetic products can induce dermatitis upon short-term use on normal skin [167, 168]. Thus, the European Union (EU) issued a Cosmetics Directive, stating that a label warning consumers of formaldehyde content must be placed on products that release a free formaldehyde concentration >0.05 % by weight (500 ppm) [169]. Moreover, Europe limits the maximum concentrations of FRP's in products as well [170].

Formaldehyde is included in the T.R.U.E. Test at site #21. In an effort to decrease sensitization by lowering formaldehyde concentrations, formaldehyde releasing preservatives (FRP's) (see #'s 35–41) were developed; however, sensitization to these chemicals continues to grow in prevalence, making FRP's a potential source of formaldehyde exposure as well [171].

Occupational exposure to formaldehyde is a risk for dermatologists, embalmers, pathologists, hemodialysis nurses, and garment industry workers.

Sources (*including formaldehyde releasing preservatives*) [18, 165, 166, 172, 173]:

Automobile: exhaust, antifreeze, rust inhibitor
Building materials

- Fiberboard
- Insulation
- Paints
- Particle board
- Plywood

Cigarette smoke

34. Formaldehyde

Cleaners: glass and metal household, rug or carpet, tire, toilet bowl, window
Clothing/Fabrics

- Corduroy
- Pre-shrunk
- Permanent press
- Polyester blends with rayon or cotton
- Rayon (spun and rayon-acetate blends)
- Screen printed
- Tanning agents (leather)
- Water, moth, mildew, and sweat-proof
- Wrinkle-resistant linen or cotton

Cosmetics (see FRP's #'s 35–41)
Cutting fluids
Deodorizers and disinfectants
Embalming fluid and fixatives
Formica – formaldehyde and urea polymer [174]
Foods containing formaldehyde [164, 175, 176] (Table 2.7):
Glues
Medical permethrin cream
Metal working fluids
Nail polish and hardeners
Paints and lacquers, including removers
Paper treating and coating
Personal hygiene products – (see FRP's #'s 35–41)

- Baby wipes
- Body wash
- Conditioners
- Cream
- Gel
- Hand soap
- Lotion
- Shampoo

Pesticides
Photographic chemicals
Plastics and resins: phenolic resins, urea plastics, polyacetal resins, melamine resins

TABLE 2.7 Foods containing formaldehyde

Dairy	Drinks	Fish	Fruits and vegetables	Miscellaneous
Italian cheese: grana cheese (hard grating)	Coffee (more so with instant coffee)	Caviar and herring from Scandinavian countries	Dried bean curd	Hydrated food
Yogurt (with aspartame)[a]	Diet soda (with aspartame)[a]	Frozen cod	Shitake mushrooms	Maple syrup
		Haddock		Smoked ham
		Pollack		Vermicelli

[a]Aspartame (Nutrasweet): Formaldehyde is a biological degradation product of aspartame through methanol oxidization

Polishes and finishes: automobile, windshield, floor, cement floor, shoe, suede shoe, furniture
Printing ink
Rubber latex – preservative and coagulant
Smog
Starch (aerosol laundry)
Vaccines

- Inactivated Polio Vaccine [177]
- Anthrax Vaccine Adsorbed [178]
- Diphtheria and Tetanus Toxoids and Acellular Pertussis Vaccine Adsorbed [179]
- Hepatitis A Vaccine (*Formalin: not more than 0.1 mg/mL*) [180]

Allergen of the Year: N/A

Degree of Relevance: High (in children as well) [18, 166, 182]

Classic Presentation: Hand dermatitis [173] and eyelid dermatitis [182], as well as other presentations related to the site of contact with the product containing the allergen. For example, in textile dermatitis, regions where clothing rubs against the skin, i.e. body folds, are affected [183].

Potential Ectopic Dermatitis: possible, given the use of formaldehyde releasing preservatives in personal care products.

Potential Generalized/Systemic Dermatitis [184, 185]: Yes. Systemic exposure to formaldehyde is possible through ingestion of certain foods that metabolize into formic acid (i.e. aspartame containing foods) [176, 186, 187] or inhalation of cigarette smoke. Improvement through dietary avoidance has been reported. In addition, ACD to formaldehyde used in clothing can present as diffuse nummular dermatitis or erythroderma [164].

Co-reactivity/Cross-reactivity: cross-reactivity to FRP, especially Quaternium-15, due the formaldehyde release, rather than the chemical [188] (see #'s 35–41). Also, there is a possible cross-reactivity with glutaraldehyde (see # 64).

Test:

Patch test
Repeat Open Application Test (ROAT)

35–41. Formaldehyde Releasing Preservatives (FRPs) [189]

Description: preservatives with both antibacterial and antifungal disinfectant properties that have largely replaced formaldehyde in biocides and personal hygiene products [48]. They are reversible polymers of formaldehyde [190] and include: **35. quaternium-15, 36. diazolidinyl urea** (Germall II), **37. DMDM hydantoin** (Glydant), **38. imidazolidinyl urea** (Germall), **39. 2-bromo-2-nitropropane-1,3-diol** (Bronopol), **40. tris nitromethane** (Tris Nitro), and **41. sodium hydroxymethylglycinate** (SHMG) [191, 192]. FRP's were initially developed with the idea that the amount of free formaldehyde released would not be sufficient to induce sensitization or cause a reaction in those already sensitized, but that antimicrobial properties would be maintained [171]. Approximately 20 % of cosmetics and personal care products in the United States contain a formaldehyde-releaser, with imidazolidinyl urea (7 %) being the most frequent [170].

Quaternium-15, however, is known to have the highest sensitization potential, possibly due to its large release of formaldehyde [173, 181]. Importantly, other quaternium compounds have not been shown to cause contact allergy. ACD is possible to formaldehyde, FRP's, or both [190]; reactions to FRP's may be caused by either the release of formaldehyde or the chemical structure itself [183, 193]. The T.R.U.E. Test currently includes four FRP's, i.e. quaternium-15 (site #18), diazolidinyl urea (site #25), imidazolidinyl urea (site #29)., and bronopol (site #36).

Occupational exposure to formaldehyde and FRP's is possible in professions such as hair dressing, painting, printing, textile dyeing, paper processing, and working with disinfectants.

Sources:

Baby wipes
Body washes
Conditioners
Construction materials

Cosmetics – blush, foundation, mascara
Creams, lotions
Hair gel
Industry – cutting fluids
Medicaments (generic corticosteroid creams)
Paints and lacquers
Paper – pigmented, packaging paper
Shampoos
Soaps, liquid

Allergen of the Year: N/A

Degree of Relevance: high [181]

Classic Presentation: Hand dermatitis; Quaternium 15 has been found to be the most common allergen in hand ACD [194]

Potential Ectopic Dermatitis: Possible

Potential Generalized/Systemic Dermatitis: Yes. (See Formaldehyde #34)

Co-reactivity/Cross-reactivity: cross-reactivity to formaldehyde or other formaldehyde-releasing preservatives, due to the formaldehyde release, rather than the chemical itself [188]. In addition, fragrances may co-react due to similar product utilization patterns.

Test:

Patch test
Repeat Open Application Test (ROAT)

42–50. Fragrance Mix I & 51–57. Fragrance Mix II, Including 58–60. Essential Oils

Description: Fragrances can be individual chemicals or complex mixtures of natural and synthetic materials used in various products to provide a particular flavor or scent [195]. Fragrance mix I (FM 1) contains 1 % concentration of eight common fragrance chemicals (**43. geraniol, 44. cinnamic aldehyde, 45. hydroxycitronellal, 46. cinnamic alcohol, 47. eugenol, 48. isoeugenol, 49. oak moss absolute, and 50. a-amylcinnamic alcohol**) and fragrance mix II contains six fragrance chemicals (**52. lyral, 53. citral, 54. citronellol, 55. farnesol, 56. coumarin, and 57. hexyl cinnamic aldehyde**); both are used to screen for fragrance allergy.

Since 1957, fragrance allergy had continually been reported in the medical literature [196], eventually creating the need for a means of identifying sensitized individuals. Therefore, in the late 1970s, Larsen [197] proposed a mixture of ingredients as a screening tool for fragrance contact allergy, which contained the eight primary substances present in the Mycolog® cream. These fragrance ingredients are what we now know of as fragrance mix I [198]. This composite, in conjunction with balsam of Peru, detects a significant proportion of fragrance allergies [199]. Fragrance mix I is included in the TRUE Test panel as #6.

Avoidance of fragrances can be challenging, as product labeling may be complicated by listing individual fragrance names without indicating "fragrance." In addition, labeling may also be inadvertently misleading, as the terms "unscented" and "fragrance-free" are not synonymous. Masking fragrances may be present in "unscented" products to eliminate odor, but result in the lack of scent. "Fragrance free," however, refers to the absence of chemicals added to enhance aroma or mask odor. Lastly, certain fragrances may be utilized for their other properties (eg: preservative or emollient properties); these 'covert fragrances' may be added without the need to disclose "fragrances" [200, 201] (see Table 2.8) [200].

TABLE 2.8 Covert fragrances

Benzyl alcohol

Bisabolol (chamomile oil)

Citrus oils

Essential oils of plants or flowers

Farnesol

Flavorings: menthol, sweet almond oil, vanilla

Maltol

Importantly, essential oils, such as **58. jasmine absolute**, **59. tea tree oil**, and **60. ylang ylang**, are also considered fragrances, and may be patch tested separately.

Sources: ubiquitous in scented products, and some "unscented" [15, 18, 77, 195]

Aftershaves
Animal by-products – ambergris, musk, civet, and castoreum
Antiseptics
Candles
Colognes
Cosmetics – concealers, eyeshadows, eyeliners, foundations, lipsticks, powders, make-up removers, nail products (quick-dry)
Chewing gums
Creams
Dental cements
Dentrifices – toothpaste, mouthwashes
Deodorants
Drinks – colas, vermouth
Essential oils
Flavorings
Foods – honey, tomatoes
Hair products – gels, mousses, shampoos
Herbicides
Household products – cleaners, detergents, room fresheners
Insecticides

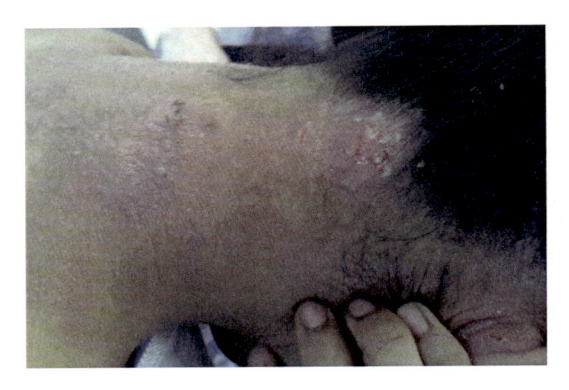

FIGURE 2.4 Allergic contact dermatitis of the posterior neck and scalp to fragrances

Lotions
Medical pastes and gels – EKG gels
Medicaments (topical)
Perfumes
Personal hygiene products – diapers, panty liners, sanitary pads, tampons, tissue, toilet paper
Plants/botanicals – cloves, sassafras
Spices – allspice, cinnamon, nutmeg
Soaps
Sunscreen

Allergen of the Year: 2007
Degree of Relevance: high
Classic Presentation: ACD of the head, neck, posterior auricular region, and face (eyelids, mouth, lips), as well as axillae and hands are common presentations [202]. Fragrance allergy also appears to predominate in women, with a female to male ratio of 3–4:1, which may be due to a greater proportion of women utilizing fragranced skin care products and perfumes [198]. In fact, on average, a perfume is composed of 30–50 chemicals used to create the particular scent [36]. Moreover, the application of perfumes to the neck region largely accounts for the classic presentation of ACD (Figs. 2.4, 2.5, and 2.6).

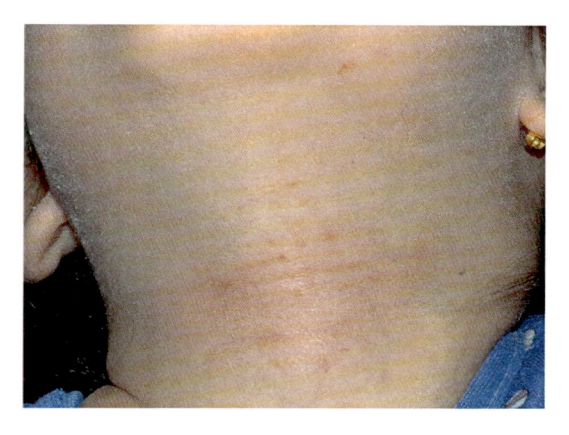

FIGURE 2.5 Allergic contact dermatitis of the anterior neck due to fragrances and neomycin in a pediatric patient

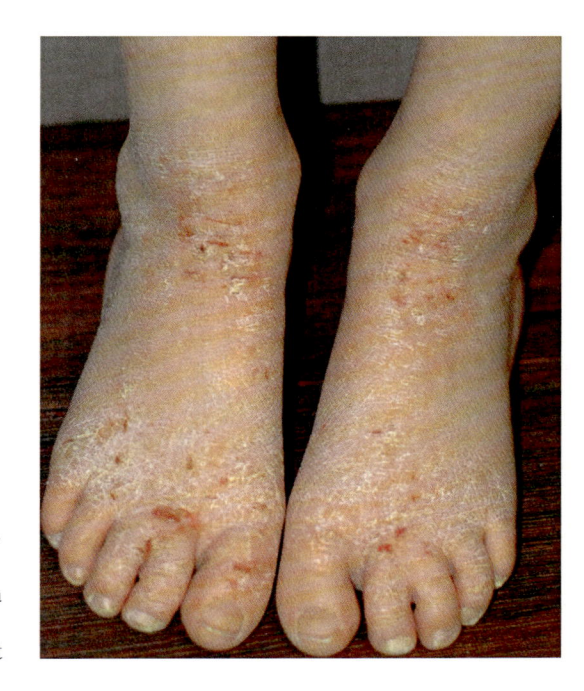

FIGURE 2.6 ACD of the feet to fragrances, lanolin and sorbitans, in a pediatric atopic patient

Oral and perioral dermatitis can be caused by the fragrances/flavorings used in toothpastes, chewing gums, mouthwashes, and mentholated cigarettes. In addition, diaper dermatitis may be due to fragrances used in the diaper itself or in products applied to the diaper region, i.e. lotions, salves [203].

"Consort" or "connubial" contact dermatitis also can occur by contact with others, such as partners, care-givers, friends or co-workers, that utilize certain products [77, 202].

Potential Ectopic Dermatitis: Yes, the eyelid can be affected by aerosolization of fragrances and then occlusion when eyes are open.

Potential Generalized/Systemic Dermatitis: Yes; Airborne contact, and systemic exposure by inhalation and ingestion of flavored foods, drinks, etc. may occur [202].

Co-reactivity/Cross-reactivity: cross-reactivity to balsam of Peru (*Myroxylon pereirae*), as some of the individuals fragrances included in FM1 are constituents of BOP (see #4).

Supplemental patch testing trays are available, such as fragrance/flavors, and specifically balsam of Peru components at some institutions [204], with the idea that by including constituents and cross-reactors of the allergen in question, the chance of detecting relevant positive reactions is greater [37].

Test:

Patch test – many products, such as creams and cosmetics, may be tested "as is"
Repeat Open Application Test (ROAT)

61–63. Gallates (Propyl, Octyl, Dodecyl)

Description: gallic acid esters used as antioxidants and often added to food or cosmetic products in order to prevent the oxidation of fats and oils, leading to spoilage. Propyl ester is more water soluble than fat soluble; however, both octyl and dodecyl esters are more fat soluble [205].

Sources: Gallates are most often found in oily, greasy, or high fat foods, as well as oily or waxy cosmetics.

Propyl Gallate:

> Antiperspirant/Deoderant
> Bar soap
> Creams
> Cosmetics
>> Concealer
>> Eye brow liner
>> Eye liner or shadow
>> Lip balm, gloss, or liner
>> Mascara
>> Powder
>
> Facial cleanser
> Foods
>> Chewing gum
>> Dry breakfast cereals
>> Meat products
>> Soup base
>> Vegetable oil/shortening
>
> Lotions
> Moisturizer
> Oils, including tanning
> Perfumes
> Shaving cream
> Sunscreen (sunblock)

Octyl Gallate:

Cosmetics (some)
Emulsion waxes
Foods and Drinks that contain octyl gallate (Table 2.9)
Transformer oils
Paints
Plastics
Polish
Varnish

Dodecyl Gallate:

Foods

Cheese
Margarine
Mayonnaise
Peanut butter

Allergen of the Year: N/A

Degree of Relevance: low; however, all three gallates are moderate to strong sensitizers, with dodecyl gallate being the strongest [205].

Classic Presentation: Dermatitis at the site of application. Lip edema and oral ulcerations have also been reported with ingestion of octyl and dodecyl gallate [205].

Potential Ectopic Dermatitis: unknown

Potential Generalized/Systemic Dermatitis: Octyl gallate has caused an airborne contact dermatitis upon heating with chicken fat [205].

Co-reactivity/Cross-reactivity: Gallates may cross-react with each other; therefore, it cannot be assumed that if a patient is allergic to one type of gallate, he or she may substitute another. Ideally, all three gallates should be tested before assigning alternative options.

Test:

Patch test
Repeat Open Application Test (ROAT)

TABLE 2.9 Foods and drinks that contain Octyl Gallate

Dairy	Drinks	Fats	Fruits	Grains/nuts	Miscellaneous
	Beer	Lard	Canned fruits	Cereal	Dairy products
		Margarine		Peanut butter	Processed meats/fish
		Mayonnaise			Snack foods
		Oils (edible)			
		Salad dressings			
		Shortening			

64. Glutaraldehyde

Description: a powerful and popular biocide with activity against a variety of bacteria, viruses, and fungi, including Human Immunodeficiency Virus (HIV) and *Mycobacterium tuberculosis*. It is, however, both an irritant as well as contact allergen, often affecting health care workers, especially in dentistry [206–208], as it is often used to sterilize medical and dental equipment. Moreover, janitorial workers can also be effected by contact with cleaning supplies. ACD due to glutaraldehyde may be persistent secondary to continued occupational use. In response to the rise in contact allergy to this chemical, the National Institute of Occupational Safety and Health (NIOSH) has published guidelines for safe handling of glutaraldehyde.

Sources [173, 194, 206]:

Disinfectants
Embalming fluids
Fabric softeners
Sterilizing solutions
Waterless hand soaps

Allergen of the Year: N/A
Degree of Relevance: high in health care fields [207]
Classic Presentation: related to site of contact, but hands often effected [206].

Potential Ectopic Dermatitis: possible, from retained products on cleaning supplies, such as mop handles

Potential Generalized/Systemic Dermatitis: possible

Co-reactivity/Cross-reactivity: Co-reactivity with formaldehyde reported, cross-reactivity reported very rarely. (see #34) [207].

Test:

Patch test
Repeat Open Application Test (ROAT)

65. Gold Sodium Thiosulfate

Description: soft, yellow, precious metal predominantly used for jewelry, currency and in electronics and dental industries. Included on the T.R.U.E. Test at site #28.

Sources [209]:

Ceramics and glassware
Currency (coins)
Dental appliances
Electronic circuits
Enamels
Food: edible gold and silver leafing and flakes for cookie decorating; Goldschläger schnapps with very thin, yet visible flakes of gold leaf in it.
Gold-plating
Jewelry
Medicines
Photography

Allergen of the Year: 2001
Degree of Relevance: low to moderate [209]
Classic Presentation: The presentation is rarely at the site of contact with jewelry, but rather involves the eyelid and mouth (stomatitis) [210, 211]. Black dermographism can also be observed, i.e. 'black writing' that appears on the skin with exposure to gold.
Potential Ectopic Dermatitis: Yes; titanium dioxide in cosmetics abrades gold particles from jewelry worn elsewhere, resulting in a facial contact dermatitis where the product is applied [212]
Potential Generalized/Systemic Dermatitis: Systemic contact dermatitis is possible albeit rare [213].
Co-reactivity/Cross-reactivity: unlikely
Test:

Patch test [granulomatous reactions may be seen]

66. Iodopropynyl Butylcarbamate (IPBC) or Glycacil

Description: broad spectrum preservative with activity against bacteria, fungi, and mites [173].

Sources: often occupational exposures, but MSDS may not be reliable to list all ingredients [100, 173]

Adhesives
After shave lotions
Baby wipes
Cosmetics, including eye makeup remover
Cutting Oils
Detergents
Face wash and masks
Hair products

- Conditioners
- Dyes
- Shampoos

Metal working fluids [214]
Moisturizers
Paints
Soaps
Tanning preparations
Textiles
Wallpaper
Wood industry

Allergen of the Year: N/A

Degree of Relevance: low; the NACDG reported 24 positive results after patch testing 5,137 patients [215]; Bryld et al. from Denmark reported 7 of 3,168 patients patch tested positive [216]; The Information Network of Departments of Dermatology (IVDK) in Germany reported 16 positive patch tests in a group of 4,883 patients, with possible false negatives suggested [217]. The testing concentration of IPBC has now been increased by the NACDG from 0.1 to 0.2 % to reduce false negative results based on recommendations from the IVDK [173, 218]

Classic Presentation: related to site of exposure; it can be responsible for hand dermatitis [173]

Potential Ectopic Dermatitis: unlikely

Potential Generalized/Systemic Dermatitis: IPBC is not used in aerosolized products due to pulmonary toxicity observed in animal models [219]

Co-reactivity/Cross-reactivity: Cross-reactivity with carbamates (see #79)

Test:

Patch test
Repeat Open Application Test (ROAT)

67. Lanolin (Wool wax Alcohol) [220–222]

Description: emollient derived from sheep sebum and used for skin barrier protection and repair, whose constituents may vary. This means that lanolin sensitized individuals may react to one lanolin preparation, but not another. Trade names include Amerchol BL, C, and H-9. Lanolin holds site #2 on the T.R.U.E Test.

Sources:

After-shave
Antiperspirant
Baby and bath oils
Corrosion inhibitors
Cosmetics – blush, chapsticks, eye shadows, lip balms, lipsticks
Creams, lotions, moisturizers, and ointments
Diaper and nursing dermatitis remedies
Hairspray
Hand sanitizers (waterless)
Hemorrhoidal remedies
Industrial products – clock and cylinder oils, cutting oils, lubricants, rust preventives, solvents
Inks
Moist towelettes
Polishes – furniture and shoe
Shampoos
Shaving cream
Soaps
Steroid, topical preparations
Sunscreens
Suntan oils
Wound care

Allergen of the Year: N/A
Degree of Relevance: high (children) [18–20, 223]
Classic Presentation: related to body sites of distribution/application, often hands (Fig. 2.7).

FIGURE 2.7 Allergic contact dermatitis of the popliteal fossa from lanolin

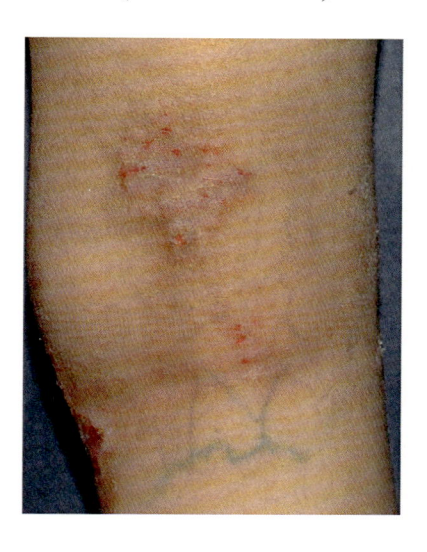

Potential Ectopic Dermatitis: unlikely
Potential Generalized/Systemic Dermatitis: unlikely
Co-reactivity/Cross-reactivity: not relevant
Test:

Patch test
Repeat Open Application Test (ROAT)

68. Methylchloroisothiazolone Methylisothiazolone (MCI/MI)

Description: a mixture of 1.15 % MCI and 0.35 % MI, marketed under Kathon CG, Euxyl K100, and Amerstat 250, and used as an effective biocide against both Gram-positive and Gram-negative bacteria, as well as fungi, at low concentrations.

Sources [100]:

Cosmetics
Industry – jet fuels, latex paint, metalworking, paper mills
Moist wipes
Shampoos

Allergen of the Year: N/A

Degree of Relevance: moderate [173, 224, 225]; Restriction on the use of MCI/MI has been initiated in Japan, by the Cosmetic Ingredient Review (based in Washington, D.C.), and by the European Economic Community, to concentrations 15 ppm or less in rinse-off products and 7.5 ppm or less in leave-on products [173], which is within the range of effectiveness [133].

Classic Presentation: based on site of contact, especially hand dermatitis, with occupational exposure one means on contact [173].

Potential Ectopic Dermatitis: unlikely
Potential Generalized/Systemic Dermatitis: unlikely
Co-reactivity/Cross-reactivity: not relevant
Test:

Patch test
Repeat Open Application Test (ROAT)

69. Methyldibromoglutaronitrile (MDBGN)

Description: preservative, often combined with **70. phenoxyethanol (PE)**, forming Euxyl K400, which is biostatic against bacteria and fungi [226]. MDBGN, however, is the most sensitizing component and the key preservative as well; it is now included on the T.R.U.E. Test at site #32 [173].

Sources [173]:

Adhesives
Cosmetics
Industrial

- Fuels
- Lubricants
- Oils
- Solvents

Latex paint
Metalworking fluids
Paper
Toilet paper (moist)

Allergen of the Year: N/A
Degree of Relevance: moderate
Classic Presentation: Hand dermatitis, often occupational [194], and facial, often due to cosmetics [227]
Potential Ectopic Dermatitis: unlikely
Potential Generalized/Systemic Dermatitis: not likely
Co-reactivity/Cross-reactivity: not likely
Test:

Patch test

71. Neomycin Sulfate

Description: topical, aminoglycoside antibiotic that for approximately 25 years, has been the second most common sensitizing allergen [228]. It has activity against Gram-negative bacilli by irreversibly inhibiting protein synthesis [229]. However, neomycin is poorly absorbed in the gastrointestinal tract, making it better suited for topical application to skin and mucous membrane infections, as well as wounds and burns [230]. Neomycin is located in site #3 of the T.R.U.E. Test.

Sources [230]:

Cosmetics – rare
Deodorants – rare
Over-the-counter medications [231] – ointments, creams, eye drops, ear drops, medicated first aid plasters: treats skin, eye, and ear infections
Pet foods
Soaps – rare
Vaccines that contain varying amounts of neomycin [232]:

- Diphtheria and tetanus toxoids and acellular pertussis adsorbed, hepatitis B recombinant and inactivated poliovirus combined
- Diphtheria and tetanus toxoids and acellular pertussis adsorbed and inactivated poliovirus
- Diphtheria and tetanus toxoids and acellular pertussis adsorbed, inactivated poliovirus and Haemophilus B conjugate
- Poliovirus, inactivated (monkey kidney cell)
- Hepatitis A, inactivated
- Hepatitis A inactivated and hepatitis B recombinant
- Influenza virus, and influenza A (H1N1) 2009 monovalent
- Influenza virus, trivalent, types A and B, and influenza A (H1N1) 2009 Monovalent
- Influenza virus, trivalent, types A and B
- Measles virus, live
- Measles, mumps, and rubella virus, live
- Measles, mumps, rubella and varicella virus, live

- Mumps virus, live
- Rubella virus, live
- Rabies

Veterinary products

Allergen of the Year: 2010

Degree of Relevance: High (The rise of bacitracin use came with a decrease in neomycin allergy prevalence in the US)

Classic Presentation: site of application, i.e. eczema sites, wounds [233]

Potential Ectopic Dermatitis: unlikely

Potential Generalized/Systemic Dermatitis: rare [234], but erythroderma has been reported after administration of gentamycin in a nickel sensitive patient [235].

Co-reactivity/Cross-reactivity: co-reactivity with bacitracin [236], (see # 3) as both allergens are often used together in topical antibiotic products. Cross-reactivity can be observed with streptomycin, gentamycin, tobramycin, kentamycin, paromomycin, butirosin, franmycetin, and ambutrosin.

Test:

Patch test
Repeat Open Application Test (ROAT)

72. Nickel Sulfate

Description: ubiquitous metal that is found in elemental form in the earth's crust, comprising about 3 % of the composition of the earth [237]. It is also the most prevalent allergen in patch tested patients of all ages [28, 238]. Nickel is widely used in metal alloys and nickel cast iron; however, when compounded with stainless steel, sensitized individuals do not develop dermatitis [239]. Interestingly, exposure of the oral mucosa to nickel prior to cutaneous sensitization has been shown to induce immune tolerance, i.e. through application of orthodontic braces [235]. Nickel holds the #1 site on the T.R.U.E. Test.

Sources [36, 240]:

Batteries (alkaline)
Cellular phones [241, 242] (Fig. 2.8)
Cigarette lighters and smoking
Clothing – jean snaps, belt buckles, zippers, buttons, suspenders
Coin money
Cosmetics – powder compacts, lipstick holders

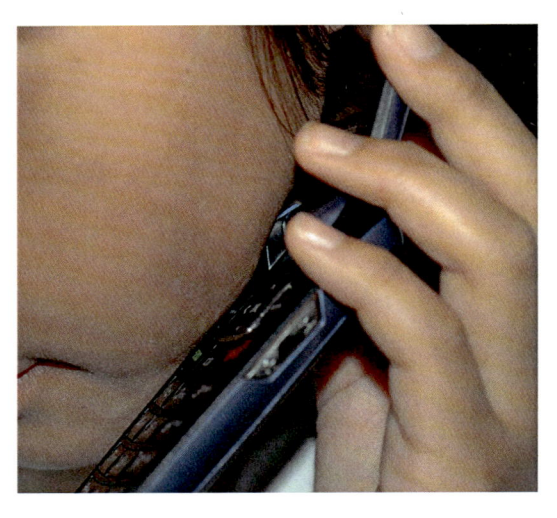

FIGURE 2.8 Facial reaction to the nickel in the cell phone

Dental appliances – orthodontia
Door knobs
Eyeglass frames
Foods containing nickel [239, 243, 244] (Table 2.10)– The average American diet contains 0.3–0.6 mg of nickel per day, with the amount of nickel in foods partially determined by the soil, fungicides, and handling equipment [237, 245].
Furniture – studs on school chairs, knobs
Jewelry [246] – including watches, earrings
Keys and key rings
Kitchen items – utensils, appliances
Music Instruments [247] – wind, guitar strings, horns
Office items – pens, paper-clips, scissors
Orthopedic materials
Razors
Tools – pliers, wrenches, screwdrivers

Allergen of the Year: 2008

Degree of Relevance: highest

Classic Presentation: relates to contact with jewelry, i.e. earlobes, neck, wrists, and from contact with jean snaps and belt buckles, i.e. infraumbilical [18] (Fig. 2.9). Vesicular palmar dermatitis has also been reported upon systemic exposure [235].

Potential Ectopic Dermatitis: Yes (reported from cell phones [248], pruritus ani [249])

Potential Generalized/Systemic Dermatitis: Yes [250]; systemic contact dermatitis, sometimes generalized, has been documented with food-related triggers [15] and inhalation [239]. The most common clinical presentation of systemic dermatitis is recurrent vesicular palmar eczema [235, 251].

Co-reactivity/Cross-reactivity: As nickel and cobalt (see #13) are often found together in nature and in metal objects, and the presumed cross-sensitivity with cobalt may be the result of concomitant sensitization [252].

Test:
Patch test

Confirmatory nickel detection testing kit, containing 1 % dimethylglyoxime-ammonia (DMG-A), which can be applied

TABLE 2.10 Foods containing nickel

Grains	Vegetables (0.093)[a]	Fruits (01.12)[a]	Nuts (10.19)[a]	Seafood (0.048)[a]	Drinks/desserts
Bran	Asparagus	Dates	Almonds	Crawfish	Baking powder
Buckwheat	Beans (green, brown, white)	Figs	Hazelnuts	Mussels	Beer
Multigrain breads (0.097)[a]	Kale	Pineapple	Peanuts (peanut butter)	Oysters	Chocolate (especially dark) (1.352)[a]
Oatmeal	Leeks	Prune		Shrimp	Cocoa
Sesame seeds	Lettuce	Raspberries			Red wine
Rice (unpolished) (0.038)[a]	Peas (green and split)				Tea (from dispensers)
	Soy protein/beans				
	Spinach				

[a] Mean concentrations (mg/kg fresh weight) are listed in parentheses

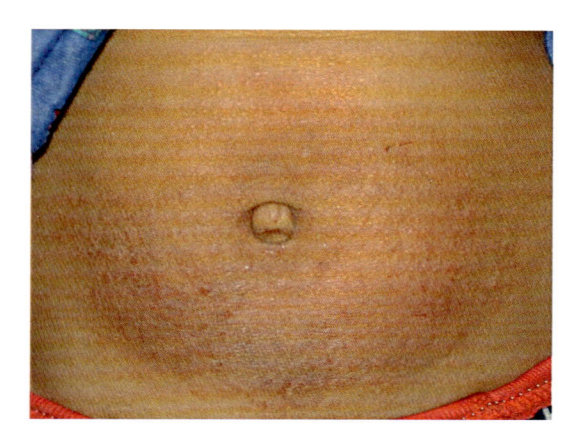

FIGURE 2.9 Peri-umbilical allergic contact dermatitis to nickel

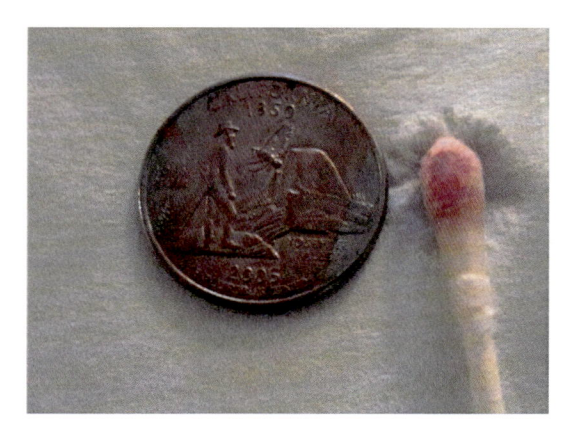

FIGURE 2.10 Positive nickel confirmatory test using 1 % dimethylglyoxime-ammonia (DMG-A), which turns pink upon contact with nickel items

to any product in question. A pink indicator color will appear on the applicator tip if the product contains nickel in a concentration of at least 1:10,000 [240] (Fig. 2.10).

73. p-Phenylenediamine (PPD)

Description: colorless aromatic amine, derived from para-aminobenzoic acid (PABA) and used as an antioxidant and initially formulated for use in hair dyes in 1907. It is itself oxidized, contributing to the black pigment of hair dyes. This led to the development of PPD derivatives for use in the automotive tire industry, which are now components of black rubber mix (see #7) [92].

Due to adverse allergic contact reactions to PPD used in mascaras, the Food, Drug, and Cosmetic Act of 1938 banned the use of PPD on skin, and later, all at-home hair dye kits were mandated to provide instructions for consumers to test themselves for sensitization [86].

Sources [36]:

Hair dye (permanent) – acts as a primary intermediate. It is oxidized by hydrogen peroxide and then polymerized to a color using a coupler, such as resorcinol. The limit permissible for hair dyes is <6 %. In the 1930's, women utilized PPD as a tinting agent for their eyelashes (mascara) and eyebrows, causing adverse reactions, some quite serious [86].

Temporary tattoos – using natural henna mixed with PPD to make 'black henna' [253, 254], potentially inducing sensitization and subsequent cutaneous reactions, including bullous type, hyper- and hypopigmentation and permanent scarring. PPD has been detected in concentrations >15 % in henna tattoo preparations [255], causing children and adolescents to become sensitized, placing them at risk for unusually severe reactions to PPD containing hair dyes [256, 257].

Allergen of the Year: 2006
Degree of Relevance: high
Classic Presentation: related to site of exposure, i.e. scalp (hairline), ears, hands, tattoo location
Potential Ectopic Dermatitis: eyelids (potential aerosolization) and hands (touching) of client getting his or her hair dyed

Potential Generalized/Systemic Dermatitis: Yes, when exposed to cross-reactors, such as benzocaine, hydrochlorothiazide, and sulfonamide medications [258, 259].

Co-reactivity/Cross-reactivity: Cross-reactivity to black rubber mix (see #7): PPD derivatives, e.g. isopropyl-paraphenylenediamine and related chemicals, are used in screening for black rubber allergy. PPD, however, is a poor detector of sensitization for black rubber allergy. Cross-reactivity is also possible to additional PABA derivatives, such as ester anesthetics (benzocaine), hydrochlorothiazide, and sulfonamide medications, as well as certain dark synthetic clothing, possibly containing semi-permanent dyes, in about 25 % of PPD allergic patients [36, 86]

Test:

Patch test

Repeat Open Application Test (ROAT)

74. p-Tert Butylphenol Formaldehyde Resin (PTBFR)

Description [260]: adhesive resin utilized in neoprene and foam, often with dialkylthioureas, together commonly referred to as 'neoprene cement' allergens.

Sources:

Cars upholstery glue

Clothing items glue/foams: bras and shoes (leather and rubber) [261]

Neoprene

Sports gear equipment (protective)

Allergen of the Year: N/A

Degree of Relevance: high

Classic Presentation: related to body site of contact/exposure, often foot and sports gear distribution

Potential Ectopic Dermatitis: unlikely

Potential Generalized/Systemic Dermatitis: unknown

Co-reactivity/Cross-reactivity: Co-reactivity with dialkyl thioureas (see #84)

Test:

Patch test

75. Paraben Mix

Description: Paraben, or para-hydroxybenzoic acid, are alkyl esters used as preservatives. The most commonly used esters are methyl-, propyl-, benzyl-, ethyl-, and butyl-paraben [173, 262]. Antimicrobial actions are greater against fungi than bacteria and greater against Gram-positive than Gram-negative bacteria [262]. Due to this, parabens are often combined with other preservatives, such as the formaldehyde releasing preservatives, in order to increase their spectrum of action.

A mix of parabens, consisting of methyl-, ethyl-, propyl-, and butyl-paraben, is initially used in patch testing to screen the patient in the United States [191]. Further testing with individual parabens is conducted if this initial screen is positive [251].

Sources [263]:

Cosmetic
Creams
Medicaments

Allergen of the Year: N/A

Degree of Relevance: low; contact allergy to parabens is low relative to its prevalence in consumer products [215, 227]

Classic Presentation: related to sites of contact with skin, especially if compromised epidermis [264]

Potential Ectopic Dermatitis: unlikely

Potential Generalized/Systemic Dermatitis: Yes; dermatitis has been reported after systemic exposure through injection of preparations preserved with parabens or oral intake [235].

Co-reactivity/Cross-reactivity: may co-react with a variety of substances, as it is used as a vehicle preservative in many products and medicaments.

Test:

Patch test
Repeat Open Application Test (ROAT)

76. Potassium Dichromate

Description: a metal salt derived from chromium.
  Sources [265]:

Cement
Ceramics
Cosmetics (green tints)
Dental appliances – implants, metal wire used in orthodontia
Dyes
Foods that contain potassium dichromate [244, 266, 267] (Table 2.11)
Green tattoo ink
Matches
Materials – green felt (pool table)
Orthopedic prostheses
Paints
Sutures (chromated catgut)
Tanned leather [268, 269] – couches, shoes, belts, gloves
Vitamin supplements

TABLE 2.11 Foods that contain potassium dichromate

Animal products	Drinks/desserts	Grains, nuts and seeds (0.27)[a]	Fruits (Fresh: 0.10; Dried: 0.27)[a]	Seafood (Crustaceans and molluscs: 0.26)[a]	Spices (0.34)[a]	Vegetables (0.12)[a] and starch
Cheese and butter (0.38–0.64)[a]	Beer (Brewer's Yeast)	High-Bran Cereals (0.28)[a]	Apple Peel	Clams	Black pepper	Baked beans
Chicken and chicken eggs (0.22–0.27)[a]	Chocolate (0.87)[a]	Wheat germ (0.14)[a]	Avocado	Cockles	Cloves	Broccoli
Liver	Cocoa	Whole grain flour (0.22)[a]	Bananas	Fish (0.24)[a]	Thyme	Corn
Liver	Ice cream, sorbets, and frozen desserts (0.36)[a]		Canned Fruits (Plums)	Mussels		Frozen or canned vegetables (frozen peas)

(continued)

TABLE 2.11 (continued)

Animal products	Drinks/desserts	Grains, nuts and seeds (0.27)[a]	Fruits (Fresh: 0.10; Dried: 0.27)[a]	Seafood (Crustaceans and molluscs: 0.26)[a]	Spices (0.34)[a]	Vegetables (0.12)[a] and starch
Processed meats (beef) (0.30–0.41)[a]	Oils and margarine (0.59–1.00)[a]		Pears	Oysters		Green beans
	Pastries and cakes (0.32)[a]		Prunes			Mushrooms
	Sugars and sugar derivatives (0.21)[a]					Onions
	Tea					Peppers (green)
	Wine					Potatoes (0.15)[a]
						Spinach
						Vegetable oil

[a]Mean Concentration (mg/kg fresh weight) in parentheses

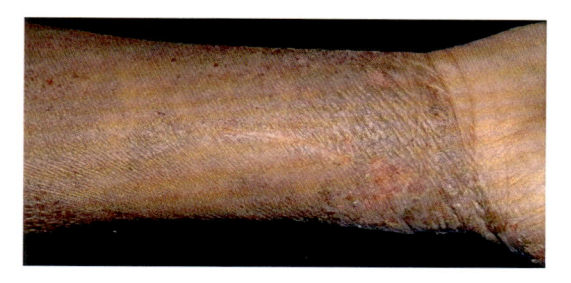

FIGURE 2.11 ACD to chromium in a construction worker

Allergen of the Year: N/A
Degree of Relevance: moderate
Classic Presentation: corresponds to body site of contact, often hands (Fig. 2.11)
Potential Ectopic Dermatitis: unlikely
Potential Generalized/Systemic Dermatitis: Yes, as worsening hand dermatitis has been documented after systemic ingestion of chromium [235].
Co-reactivity/Cross-reactivity: Potential co-reactivity with nickel and cobalt
Test:

Patch test
Repeat Open Application Test (ROAT) – cosmetic products and orthopedic test discs

77. Propylene Glycol

Description: preservative and moisture agent
 Sources:

Automotive – antifreeze, brake fluid
Antiperspirants
Baby products – lotions, creams, towelettes
Cosmetics
Foods and Drinks containing propylene glycol (Table 2.12)
Gels – EKG, transcutaneous nerve stimulator
Household products and cleaners
Inks
Ophthalmic preparations
Oral medications – cough preparations
Otic preparations
Personal care products
Plasticizers
Topical pharmaceuticals – creams, ointments (some topical anesthetics, corticosteroids, and antibiotics)

Allergen of the Year: N/A
Degree of Relevance: moderate
Classic Presentation: Face, perioral, in sites of dermatitis
Potential Ectopic Dermatitis: not likely
Potential Generalized/Systemic Dermatitis: Yes, oral ingestion of propylene glycol has been shown to cause systemic dermatitis [270].
Co-reactivity/Cross-reactivity: Co-reactivity with topical anesthetics, corticosteroids, and antibiotics.
Test:

Patch test
Repeat Open Application Test (ROAT)

Table 2.12 Foods and drinks containing propylene glycol

Desserts	**Dressings**	**Drinks**	**Miscellaneous**
Cake mixes and toppings	Cole slaw	Some sodas	Butter-flavored popcorn
Moist cakes	Salad dressing		French fried onion

78. Quinoline Mix

Description: This mix contains both clioquinol (Vioform) and chloquinaldol; quinolines are used as both antibacterial and antifungal agents. Quinoline mix is included in the T.R.U.E. Test at site #26.

Sources:

Bag Balm® ointment
Medications – topical antibiotic and antifungal creams, lotions, ointments, and bandages

Allergen of the Year: N/A
Degree of Relevance: low
Classic Presentation: relates to the region on contact.
Potential Ectopic Dermatitis: unlikely
Potential Generalized/Systemic Dermatitis: unlikely
Co-reactivity/Cross-reactivity: potential cross-reactivity with fluoroquinolones
Test:

Patch test
Repeat Open Application Test (ROAT)

79–84. Rubber Accelerators: Carbamate, Carba mix, Thiuram, Mercaptobenzothiazole, Mercapto mix, Mixed Diakyl Thioureas (Diethylthiourea and Dibutylthiourea)

Description: Rubber accelerators are additives used in the vulcanization of rubber in order to accelerate the transformation of latex from a liquid to a solid, heat-stable, durable, elastic state [271–273]. Rubber is derived from a milky fluid called latex that is produced by *Hevea brasiliensis*, the rubber tree. This natural rubber latex (NRL) provides both strength and elasticity [88] and currently, is largely supplied by Indonesia, Malaysia, Thailand, and South America. The classic, immediate, type-I hypersensitivity reaction associated with latex is due to an IgE-mediated response to the proteins within the latex, and is different from the type-IV delayed hypersensitivity reaction observed with ACD [274]. Contact allergy to various rubber accelerators in a multitude of products has been noted over decades in both adults and children, such as in regards to shoe-associated contact dermatitis [27, 275]. The moist, occluded environment created by shoes increases the risk of developing allergen sensitization and eventual dermatitis. While socks provide some barrier to chemical exposure, they do not provide complete protection, as chemicals may leach out of the shoe into the sock with continued wear.

Testing/screening for *carbamate* allergy can be accomplished using *carba mix*, which contains 1,3-diphenylguanidine (DPG), bis-(diethyldithiocarbamate) zinc (ZDC), and bis-(dibutyldithiocarbamate) zinc (ZBC); it is located at site #15 on the T.R.U.E. Test.

Mercaptobenzothiazole is also included on the T.R.U.E. Test at site #19. *Mercapto mix* (site #22) contains mercaptobenzothiazole, n-cyclohexylbenzothiazylsulfenamide (CBS), dibenzothiazyldisulfide (MBTS), and morpholinylmercaptobenzothiazole (MDR).

Thiuram mix (T.R.U.E. Test site #24) contains four *thiuram*-containing chemicals, i.e. tetramethylthiuram disulfide (TMTD), tetramethylthiuram monosulfide (TMTM), tetraethylthiuram disulfide (TETD or disulfiram), and dipentamethylenethiuram disulfide (PTD).

Mixed dialkyl thiroureas (diethylthiourea and dibutylthiourea) are used as fixative agents in photography and in production of synthetic rubber, such as neoprene

Sources [27, 276–279]: most rubber products/items

Adhesives
Balloons
Carpet backing (anti-slip)
Caulking and putty
Cements – plastic, rubber, shoe, thermoplastic, tile, waterproofing
Condoms, dental dams, and diaphragms
Cosmetic applicators and sponges
Diapers – "Lucky Luke" allergic contact dermatitis, presenting in a unique pattern reminiscent of a cowboy's gun belt holster, i.e. the hips and outer buttocks [280, 281]. The rubber accelerators, such as MBT, are implicated due to their inclusion in the elastic waist and legs of many disposable diapers [76].
Ear phones
Elastic and elastic waistbands – Bleached rubber syndrome describes the presentation of ACD that ensues when elastic waistbands containing carbamates are washed with bleach, creating a new chemical by-product with increased antigenicity [282] (Fig. 2.12).
Electric cords
Erasers
Gardening – hoses
Greases (heavy duty)
Industrial uses: anti-corrosive agents, antifreeze, automobile hoses, conveyer belts, cutting oils; lining of fuel tanks; shock absorbers
Mats

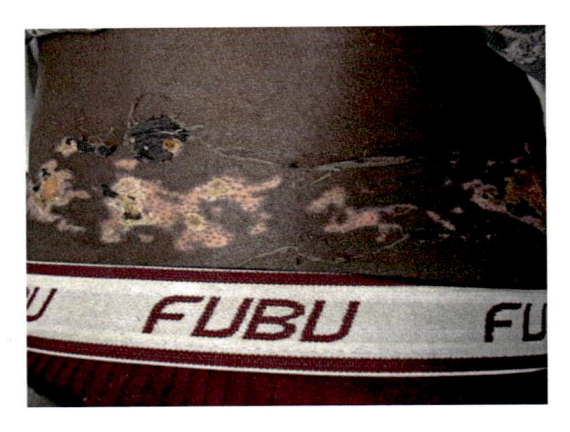

FIGURE 2.12 Bleached rubber syndrome – reaction to carbamates after bleaching underwear

Mattresses
Medical equipment – gloves [examination, surgical, household (especially thiuram)]; goggles (safety and swimming); masks (continuous positive airway pressure (CPAP) and gas); stethoscopes, tubing
Medications (Antabuse or disulfiram) [283]
Neoprene – automobile hoses, fan belt, gaskets; shin guards; swimming goggles; wetsuits
Pacifiers
Pesticides, herbicides, fungicides, seed protectant
Photographic film emulsion, fixing agents
Repellants (rabbit, rat, deer, meadow mice)
Rubber bands, sheets, and handles – tools, bicycles, toothbrushes, tennis rackets, golf clubs
Rubber in clothing – bras, girdles, shoes (including insoles and soles as well as glues, i.e. athletic shoes, boots, slippers), socks, support stockings, swimwear
Spandex (bicycle racer shorts, leotards, tights, stretch jeans, jogging suits, pantyhose, undergarments, swimwear,

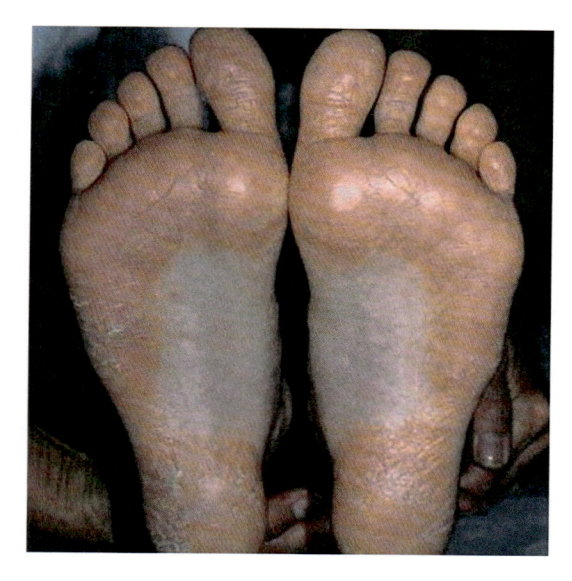

FIGURE 2.13 Allergic contact dermatitis to mercaptobenzothiazole

skiwear)- MBT and thiuram have been implicated as the primary contact allergens [27, 284, 285].
Tires
Toys and balls
Veterinary tick and flea sprays and powders

Allergen of the Year: Mixed Dialkyl Thioureas in 2009
Degree of Relevance: moderate to high
Classic Presentation: related to site of contact, often waistline, feet, and hands [278] (Fig. 2.13 and 2.14).
Potential Ectopic Dermatitis: unlikely
Potential Generalized/Systemic Dermatitis: unlikely
Co-reactivity/Cross-reactivity: Co-reactivity with thiuram, carbamate, mercaptobenzothiazole, mercapto mix, and diakylthioureas and cross-reactivity with thiuram, carbamate, and iodopropynyl butyl carbamate (see #66)

FIGURE 2.14 Allergic contact dermatitis to shin guards – dialkylthiourea component

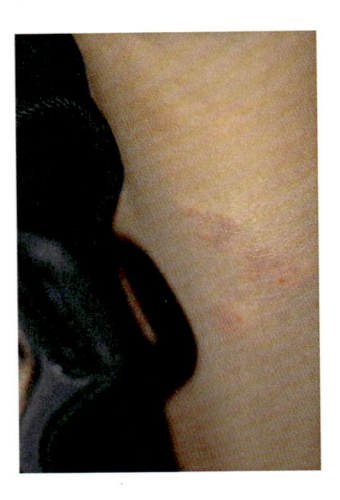

Test:

Patch test
Extraction of thiuram by testing products with acetone and cuprous acetate, looking for a color change from blue to mint green to dark green, which indicates a positive reaction [27].

85–86. Sorbitan Sesquioleate (SS) and Sorbic Acid

Description: Sorbitan sesquioleate is a fatty acid ester that is used as a water-in-oil emulsifier. It is derived from a mix of oleic acid with sorbitol.

Sources [286]:

Baby items – diaper creams, oils and lotions
Cosmetics – blush, concealer, foundation, lip balm, lip gloss, lipstick, mascara, powder
Inks and paints
Personal care products – cleansers, creams, eye makeup removers, lotions, ointments, sunscreens
Medicaments – such as topical corticosteroids [287], as well as other creams, lotions, and ointments

Allergen of the Year: N/A

Degree of Relevance: moderate, within the atopic population due to its use in corticosteroids, and recently in the pediatric population [223]

Classic Presentation: related to site of contact/application, often dermatitic sites

Potential Ectopic Dermatitis: unlikely

Potential Generalized/Systemic Dermatitis: unknown

Co-reactivity/Cross-reactivity: Potential co-reactivity with corticosteroids (see #'s 23–25). Possible cross-reactivity with related emulsifiers, Span 20 (sorbitan monolaurate), Span 40 (sorbitan monopalmitate), Span 60 (sorbitan monostearate), Span 65 (sorbitan tristearate), Span 80 (sorbitan monooleate), and Span 85 (sorbitan trioleate) [223]. **86. Sorbic acid** is a related compound with which SS may cross-react; both the acid and its salts, such as sodium sorbate, potassium sorbate, and calcium sorbate, are antimicrobial agents often used as preservatives in food and drinks.

Test:

Patch test
Repeat Open Application Test (ROAT)

87. Thimerosal

Description: preservative and disinfectant that is a mercuric derivative of thiosalicylic acid. It is also known as "tincture of Merthiolate," a first-aid product also containing ethylenediamine (see #32) and fluorescin and eosin dyes. Thimerosal is included in the T.R.U.E. Test at site #23.

Sources [288]:

Cleansers (soap-free)
Contact lens solutions
Cosmetics – eye makeup remover, mascara, bleaching creams [289]
Hormone injections
Nasal preparations/sprays
Ophthalmic medicaments, suspensions and solutions [18, 290]
Otic medicaments
Tattoo Inks – cinnabar (mercuric sulfide) [291]; manufacturers of inks and pigments, however, are not required to reveal the ingredients, as the information is proprietary.
Topical medications, anti-fungals, antiseptic sprays such as Merchromine
Vaccines – inactivated influenza vaccine is the only vaccine recommended for children below 7 years of age that still contains thimerosal [15, 290]. Adult vaccines still with this at a concentration of 0.01 % or less, in single- and/or multi-dose forms, include [232]:

- Tetanus toxoid
- Tetanus toxoid adsorbed
- Diphtheria and tetanus toxoids adsorbed
- Diphtheria and tetanus toxoids and acellular pertussis adsorbed
- Hepatitis A inactivated and hepatitis B recombinant
- Influenza virus, and influenza A (H1N1) 2009 monovalent
- Influenza virus, trivalent, types A and B, and influenza A (H1N1) 2009 monovalent
- Japanese encephalitis virus inactivated
- Meningococcal polysaccharide, groups A, C, Y and W-135 combined

Allergen of the Year: Non-Allergen of the Year, as thimerosal allergy, while common, is rarely relevant

Degree of Relevance: low; thimerosal may also be a cause of false positive patch test reactions, possibly related to prior vaccination experience.

Classic Presentation: peri-ocular

Potential Ectopic Dermatitis: Not likely

Potential Generalized/Systemic Dermatitis:

Co-reactivity/Cross-reactivity: thimerosal potentially may cross-react with inorganic ammoniated mercury. This has been controversial.

Test:

Patch test
Repeat Open Application Test (ROAT)

88. Tosylamide Formaldehyde Resin or Toluenesulfonamide Formaldehyde Resin (TSFR)

Description: a hard, practically colorless material with a faint formaldehyde odor used in nail lacquers and other nail preparations to impart high gloss and flexibility [292, 293].

Sources:

Nail lacquer
Nail preparations

Allergen of the Year: N/A

Degree of Relevance: high, responsible for most contact allergy to nail polish. The allergen is the actual resin as opposed to the formaldehyde content, as there is only a small amount of free formaldehyde present in the resin [292]. The prevalence of ACD to TSFR has decreased in recent years given the introduction of toluenesulfonamide formaldehyde resin-free nail varnishes [294].

Classic Presentation: Eyelid, peri-oral, and neck regions are often affected.

Potential Ectopic Dermatitis: Yes, ACD to this resin often occurs at sites at which that fingernails have come into contact, such as the eyelids, mouth, neck and genitalia [29].

Potential Generalized/Systemic Dermatitis: unlikely

Co-reactivity/Cross-reactivity: Doubtful formaldehyde cross-reactivity as most patients are allergic to the tosylamide resin.

Test:

Patch test with the allergen and also with the resin or dried nail lacquer

References

1. Fisher AA. Contact dermatitis. Philadelphia: LEA and Febiger; 1967. p. 5.
2. Fernández Vozmediano JM, Armario Hita JC. Allergic contact dermatitis in children. J Eur Acad Dermatol Venereol. 2005;19(1):42–6.
3. Fisher AA. Childhood allergic contact dermatitis. Cutis. 1975;15:635.
4. Mark BJ, Slavin RG. Allergic contact dermatitis. Med Clin North Am. 2006;90(1):169–85.
5. Zug KA, McGinley-Smith D, Jacob SE, Brod B, Crawford GH. Clinically relevant patch test reactions in children – a United States based study. Pediatr Dermatol. 2008;25(5):520.
6. der de Waard-van Spek FB, Oranje AP. Patch tests in children with suspected allergic contact dermatitis: a prospective study and review of the literature. Dermatology. 2009;218(2):119–25.
7. Jacob SE, Steele T. Contact dermatitis and workforce economics. Semin Cutan Med Surg. 2006;25(2):105–9.
8. American Contact Dermatitis Society. Updated 2009. http://www.contactderm.org/files/members/CoreSeries10-27-09.pdf. Accessed June 2012.
9. Perfumes, Flavors. allergEAZE allergens. Updated June 2012. http://www.allergeaze.com/allergens.aspx?ID=PF. Accessed May 2012.
10. Cosmetic Grouping. allergEAZE allergens. Updated June 2012. http://www.allergeaze.com/allergens.aspx?ID=Cosmetic. Accessed May 2012.
11. Dental Materials. allergEAZE allergens. Updated June 2012. http://www.allergeaze.com/allergens.aspx?ID=DM. Accessed May 2012.
12. Bakery Series. Chemotechnique diagnostics, p. 32–3. 2012. http://www.chemotechnique.se/Online-Catalogue.htm. Accessed June 2012.
13. Riemann H, Schwarz T, Grabbe S. Pathomechanisms of the elicitation phase of allergic contact dermatitis. J Dtsch Dermatol Ges. 2003;1(8):613–9.

14. Janeway C, Travers P, Walport M, Shlomchik M. Immunobiology: the immune system in health and disease. 6th ed. New York: Garland Science Publishing; 2005.
15. Nijhawen RI, Matiz C, Jacob SE. Contact dermatitis: from basics to allergodromes. Pediatr Ann. 2009;38(2):99–108.
16. Militello G, Jacob SE, Crawford GH. Allergic contact dermatitis in children. Curr Opin Pediatr. 2006;18:385–90.
17. Elsaie ML, Olasz E, Jacob SE. Cytokines and langerhans cells in allergic contact dermatitis. G Ital Dermatol Venereol. 2008;143(3):195–205.
18. Jacob SE, Breithaupt A. Environmental exposures – a pediatric perspective on allergic contact dermatitis. Skin Aging. 2009;17(7):28–36.
19. Zug KA, McGinley-Smith D, Warshaw EM, Taylor JS, Rietschel RL, Maibach HI, Belsito DV, Fowler Jr JF, Storrs FJ, DeLeo VA, Marks Jr JG, Mathias CG, Pratt MD, Sasseville D. Contact allergy in children referred for patch testing North American Contact Dermatitis Group data, 2001–2004. Arch Dermatol. 2008;144(10):1329–36.
20. Hogeling M, Pratt M. Allergic contact dermatitis in children: the Ottawa hospital patch-testing clinic experience, 1996 to 2006. Dermatitis. 2008;19(2):86–9.
21. Hsu J, Jacob SE. The other side of athletic safety gear in adolescents: the role of p-tert-butylphenol-formaldehyde-resin in allergic contact dermatitis. J Dermatol Nurs. 2009;1(3):198–200.
22. Vincenzi C, Guerra I, Peluso AM, Zucchelli V. Allergic contact dermatitis due to phenol-formaldehyde resin in a knee-guard. Contact Dermatitis. 1992;27(1):54.
23. Sommer S, Wilkinson SM, Dodman B. Contact dermatitis due to urea-formaldehyde resin in shin-pads. Contact Dermatitis. 1999;40(3):159–60.
24. Shono M, Ezoe K, Kaniwa M, et al. Allergic contact dermatitis from *para*-tertiary-butylphenol formaldehyde resin (PTBP-FR) in athletic tape and leather adhesive. Contact Dermatitis. 1991;24(4):281–8.
25. Azurdia RM, King CM. Allergic contact dermatitis due to phenol-formaldehyde resin and benzoyl peroxide in swimming goggles. Contact Dermatitis. 1998;38(4):234–5.
26. Herro EM, Jacob SE. Product allergen watch: p-tert-butylphenol formaldehyde resin and the impact on children. Dermatitis. 2012;23(2):86–8.
27. Rietschel RL, Fowler JF, editors. Fisher's contact dermatitis. 5th ed. Philadelphia: Lippincott Williams & Wilkins; 2001.
28. Jacob SE, Burk CJ, Connelly EA. Patch testing: another steroid-spearing agent to consider in children. Pediatr Dermatol. 2008;25(1):81–7.
29. Jacob SE, Stechschulte SA. Tosylamide/formaldehyde resin allergy – a consideration in the atopic toddler. Contact Dermatitis. 2008;58(5):312–3.

30. Jacob SE, Steele T, Brod B, Crawford GH. Dispelling the myths behind pediatric patch testing – experience from our tertiary care patch testing centers. Pediatr Dermatol. 2008;25(3):296–300.
31. Mydlarski PR, Katz AM, Mamelak AJ, et al. Contact dermatitis. In: Adkinson NF, Yunginger JW, Busse WW, editors. Middleton's allergy principles and practice. Philadelphia: Mosby; 2003. p. 1581–93.
32. Friedlander SF. Consultation with the specialist: contact dermatitis. Pediatr Rev. 1998;19(5):166–71.
33. Amaro C, Goossens A. Immunological occupational contact urticaria and contact dermatitis from proteins: a review. Contact Dermatitis. 2008;58:67–75.
34. Hjorth N, Roed-Peterson J. Occupational protein contact dermatitis in food handlers. Contact Dermatitis. 1976;2:28–42.
35. Janssens V, Morren M, Dooms-Goossens A, Degreef H. Protein contact dermatitis: myth or reality? Br J Dermatol. 1995;132:1–6.
36. Jacob SE, Herro EM, Taylor JS. Contact dermatitis: diagnosis and therapy. In: Elzouki AY, editor. Textbook of clinical pediatrics, vol. 3, Section 9. 2nd ed. Berlin, Heidelberg: Springer; 2012. p. 1467–76.
37. Nijhawan RI, Jacob SE. Patch testing: the whole in addition to the sum of its parts is greatest. Dermatitis. 2009;20(1):58–9.
38. Worm M, Aberer W, Agathos M, Becker D, Brasch J, Fuchs T, Hillen U, Hoger P, Mahler V, Schnuch A, Szliska C. Patch testing in children – recommendations of the German Contact Dermatitis Research Group (DKG). J Dtsch Dermatol Ges. 2007;5:107–9.
39. Matiz C, Russell K, Jacob SE. The importance of checking for delayed reactions in pediatric patch testing. Pediatr Dermatol. 2011;28(1):12–4.
40. Jensen CD, Paulsen E, Andersen KE. Retrospective evaluation of the consequence of alleged patch test sensitization. Contact Dermatitis. 2006;55(1):30–5.
41. Bygum A, Andersen KE. Persistent reactions after patch testing with TRUE test panels 1 and 2. Contact Dermatitis. 1998;38:218–20.
42. Wilkinson SM, Pollock B. Patch test sensitization after use of the compositae mix. Contact Dermatitis. 1999;40:277–8.
43. Devos SA, Van Der Valk PG. The risk of active sensitization to PPD. Contact Dermatitis. 2001;44:273–5.
44. Barros MA, Baptista A, Correia TM, et al. Patch testing in children: a study of 562 school children. Contact Dermatitis. 1991;25:156–9.
45. ACDS CAMP. American Contact Dermatitis Society. 2011. http://www.contactderm.org/i4a/pages/index.cfm?pageid=3489. Accessed 24 Mar 2011.
46. CARD: Contact Allergen Replacement Database. 2011. http://www.preventice.com/card/. Accessed 24 Mar 2011.
47. Jacob SE, Castanedo-Tardan MP. Pharmacotherapy for allergic contact dermatitis. Expert Opin Pharmacother. 2007;8(16):2757–74.

48. Scheman A, Jacob S, Zirwas M, Warshaw E, Nedorost S, Katta R, Cook J, Castanedo-Tardan MP. Contact allergy: alternatives for the 2007 North American Contact Dermatitis Group (NACDG) standard screening tray. Dis Mon. 2008;54(1–2):7–156.
49. Scheman A, Jacob S, Katta R, Nedorost S, Warshaw E, Zirwas M, Cha C. Part 1 of a 4-part series facial cosmetics: trends and alternatives: data from the American Contact Alternatives Group. J Clin Aesthet Dermatol. 2011;4(6):25–30.
50. Scheman A, Jacob S, Kaita R, Nedorost S, Warshaw E, Zirwas M, Bhinder M. Part 2 of a 4-part series hair products: trends and alternatives: data from the American Contact Alternatives Group. J Clin Aesthet Dermatol. 2011;4(7):42–6.
51. Scheman A, Jacob S, Katta R, Nedorost S, Warshaw E, Zirwas M, Kruk A. Part 3 of a 4-part series Lip and common dental care products: trends and alternatives: data from the American Contact Alternatives Group. J Clin Aesthet Dermatol. 2011;4(9):50–3.
52. Scheman A, Jacob S, Katta R, Nedorost S, Warshaw E, Zirwas M, Selbo N. Part 4 of a 4-part series miscellaneous products: trends and alternatives in deodorants, antiperspirants, sunblocks, shaving products, powders, and wipes: data from the American Contact Alternatives Group. J Clin Aesthet Dermatol. 2011;4(10):35–9.
53. Cohen DE, Heidary N. Treatment of irritant and allergic contact dermatitis. Dermatol Ther. 2004;17:334–40.
54. Hengge UR, Ruzicka T, Schwartz RA, Cork MJ. Adverse effects of topical glucocorticosteroids. J Am Acad Dermatol. 2006;54:1–15; quiz 6–8.
55. Marks R. Adverse side effects from the use of topical corticosteroids. In: Maibach HI, Surger C, editors. Topical corticosteroids. Basel: Karger; 1992. p. 170–83.
56. Belsito D, Wilson DC, Warshaw E, Fowler J, Ehrlich A, Anderson B, et al. A prospective randomized clinical trial of 0.1 % tacrolimus ointment in a model of chronic allergic contact dermatitis. J Am Acad Dermatol. 2006;55:40–6.
57. Wollina U. The role of topical calcineurin inhibitors for skin diseases other than atopic dermatitis. Am J Clin Dermatol. 2007;8(3):157–73.
58. Sidbury R, Hanifin JM. Systemic therapy of atopic dermatitis. Clin Exp Dermatol. 2000;25:559–66.
59. Zirwas MJ. Acrylates. Dermatitis. 2006;17(2):109–10.
60. Bjorkner B. Plastic materials. In: Adams RM, editor. Occupational skin disease. Philadelphia: WB Saunders; 1999. p. 434–64.
61. Bjorkner B. Acrylic resins. In: Kanerva I, Elsner P, Wahberg JE, Maibach HI, editors. Handbook of occupational dermatology. Berlin: Springer; 2000. p. 562–9.
62. Pratt MD, Belsito DV, DeLeo VA, et al. North American Contact Dermatitis Group patch-test results, 2001–2002 study period. Dermatitis. 2004;15:176–83.

63. Cronin H, Mowad C. Anaphylactic reaction to bacitracin ointment. Cutis. 2009;83(3):127.
64. Herro EM, Jacob SE. Allergen focus: allergic contact cheilitis. Skin Aging. 2011;19(8):18–22.
65. Jacob SE, Herro EM. Allergen focus: fragrances and flavorants. Skin Aging. 2011;19(7):23–8.
66. Chatard H. Sensitization to perfumes with skin & general reactions. Lyon Med. 1957;89(36):212–3.
67. Hjorth N. Eczematous allergy to balsams, allied perfumes and flavouring agents, with special reference to balsam of Peru. Acta Derm Venereol Suppl (Stockh). 1961;41 Suppl 46:1–216.
68. Tomar J, Jain VK, Aggarwal K, Dayal S, Gupta S. Contact allergies to cosmetics: testing with 52 cosmetic ingredients and personal products. J Dermatol. 2005;32:951–5.
69. Fisher AA. Cosmetic dermatitis in childhood. Cutis. 1995;55:15–6.
70. Salam TN, Fowler JF. Balsam-related systemic contact dermatitis. J Am Acad Dermatol. 2001;45(3):377–81.
71. Srivastava D, Cohen DE. Identification of the constituents of balsam of Peru in tomatoes. Dermatitis. 2009;20(2):99–105.
72. Magnusson B, Wilkinson DS. Cinnamic aldehyde in toothpaste. Contact Dermatitis. 1975;1:70–6.
73. Strauss RM, Orton DI. Allergic contact cheilitis in the United Kingdom: a retrospective study. Am J Contact Dermat. 2003;14:75–7.
74. Veien NK, Hattel T, Justesen O, Nørholm N. Oral challenge with balsam of Peru. Contact Dermatitis. 1985;12(2):104–7.
75. Scheinman PL. Allergic contact dermatitis to fragrance: a review. Am J Contact Dermat. 1996;7(2):65–76.
76. Herro EM, Jacob SE. Diaper dermatitis. In: Heymann WR, et al., editors. Clinical decision support: dermatology. Anticipated Publication; Fall 2012. Online publication: Copyright © 2013, Decision Support in Medicine, LLC. http://www.decisionsupportinmedicine.com/.
77. de Groot AC, Frosch PJ. Adverse reactions to fragrances. A clinical review. Contact Dermatitis. 1997;36(2):57–86.
78. Belsito DV. Surviving on a balsam-restricted diet: cruel and unusual punishment or medically necessary therapy? J Am Acad Dermatol. 2001;45(3):470–1.
79. Rietschel R, Fowler JF. Fisher's contact dermatitis. 6th ed. Hamilton: BC Decker Inc; 2008. p. 176, 417–8, 714.
80. Stanford D, Georgouras K. Allergic contact dermatitis from benzalkonium chloride in plaster of Paris. Contact Dermatitis. 1996;35(6):371–2.
81. Staniforth P. Allergy to benzalkonium chloride in plaster of Paris after sensitisation to cetrimide. A case report. J Bone Joint Surg Br. 1980;62-B(4):500–1.
82. Rietschel R, Fowler JF. Fisher's contact dermatitis. 6th ed. Hamilton: BC Decker Inc; 2008. p. 279.

83. Le Coz CJ, Bottlaender A, Scrivener JN, Santinelli F, Cribier BJ, Heid E, Grosshans EM. Photocontact dermatitis from ketoprofen and tiaprofenic acid: cross-reactivity study in 12 consecutive patients. Contact Dermatitis. 1998;38(5):245–52.
84. Jacob SE. 2006. Focus on T.R.U.E.test allergen #19 mercaptobenzothiazole & #22 mercapto mix. Skin Aging. 2006;14(9).
85. Menne T, White IR, Bruynzeel DP, Dooms-Goossens A. Patch test reactivity to the PPD-black rubber mix (industrial rubber chemicals) and individual ingredients. Contact Dermatitis. 1992; 26(5):354.
86. Jacob SE, Caperton CV. Focus on T.R.U.E. test allergen #16: black rubber mix. Skin Aging. 2006;13(6):20–4.
87. Schwartz L, Tulipan L, Birmingham DJ. Dermatoses in the manufacture of rubber. In: Occupational diseases of the skin. Philadelphia: Lea & Febiger; 1957.
88. Warshaw E. Latex allergy. Skinmed. 2003;2(6):359–66.
89. Conde-Salazar L, Del Rio E, Guimaraens D, Gonzalez Domingo A. Type IV allergy to rubber additives: a 10 year study of 686 cases. J Am Acad Dermatol. 1993;29:176–80.
90. Anderson ME, Kirkland KH, Guidotti TL, Rose C. A case study of tire crumb use on playgrounds: risk analysis and communication when major clinical knowledge gaps exist. Environ Health Perspect. 2006;114(1):1–3.
91. Weinberger LN, Seraly MP, Zirwas MJ. Palmar dermatitis due to a rubber escalator railing. Contact Dermatitis. 2006;54:59.
92. Nethercott JR, et al. Patch testing with a routine screening tray in North America, 1985–1989: gender and response. Am J Contact Dermat. 1991;2:130.
93. Jacob SE, Patel A. Focus on T.R.U.E. test allergen #5: caines. Skin Aging. 2005;13(7):22–4.
94. Rietschel R, Fowler JF. Fisher's contact dermatitis. 6th ed. Hamilton: BC Decker Inc; 2008. p. 288–95.
95. Carazo JL, Morera BS, Colom LP, Gálvez Lozano JM. Allergic contact dermatitis from ethyl chloride and benzocaine. Dermatitis. 2009;20(6):E13–5.
96. Rietschel RL, Fowler JF. Local anesthetics and topical analgesics. In: Fisher's contact dermatitis. 5th ed. New York: Lippincott Williams & Wilkins; 2001. p. 193–202.
97. Sidhu SK, Shaw S, Wilkinson JD. A 10-year retrospective study on benzocaine allergy in the United Kingdom. Am J Contact Dermat. 1999;10:57–61.
98. Rietschel R, Fowler JF. Fisher's contact dermatitis. 6th ed. Hamilton: BC Decker Inc; 2008. p. 239–53.
99. Brant WT, editor. The metallic alloys: a practical guide for the manufacture of all kinds of alloys, amalgams, and solders, used by metalworkers: together with their chemical and physical properties and their application in the arts and the industries. London: Henry Cary Baird & Co.; 1896.

100. Marks Jr JG, Elsner P, DeLeo V. Standard allergens. In: Marks Jr JG, Elsner P, DeLeo V, editors. Contact and occupational dermatology. 3rd ed. St. Louis: Mosby; 2002. p. 65–139.
101. Veien NK, Hattel T, Justesen O, Nørholm A. Oral challenge with metal salts. (I). Vesicular patch-test-negative hand eczema. Contact Dermatitis. 1983;9:402–10.
102. Stuckert J, Nedorost S. Low-cobalt diet for dyshidrotic eczema patients. Contact Dermatitis. 2008;59(6):361–5.
103. Thyssen JP, Menné T, Johansen JD, Lidén C, Julander A, Møller P, Jellesen MS. A spot test for detection of cobalt release – early experience and findings. Contact Dermatitis. 2010;63(2):63–9.
104. EM Quant® cobalt test strips. Updated 2012. http://www.emdmillipore.com/chemicals/em-quant-cobalt-test-strips/EMD_CHEM-10002/p_JvSb.s1LxioAAAEWh.IfVhTl. Accessed 15 July 2012.
105. Cobalt test strips 10–1000 ppm EM Quant. Updated 2012. http://www.galladechem.com/catalog/emd_teststrips/cobalt-test-strips-10-1000-ppm-em-quant-1-pk-of-100.htm Accessed 15 July 2012.
106. Jacob SE, Yang A, Herro EM, Zhang C. Contact allergens in a pediatric population: association with atopic dermatitis and comparison with other North American referral centers. J Clin Aesthet Dermatol. 2010;3(10):29–35.
107. Jacob SE, Amini S. Focus on allergen of the year 2004: CAPB. Skin Aging. 2006;14(8):12–4.
108. Suuronen K, Pesonen M, Aalto-Korte K. Occupational contact allergy to cocamidopropyl betaine and its impurities. Contact Dermatitis. 2012;66(5):286–92.
109. de Groot AC, van der Walle HB, Weyland JW. Contact allergy to cocamidopropyl betaine. Contact Dermatitis. 1995;33:419–22.
110. Fowler JF, Fowler LM, Hunter JE. Allergy to cocamidopropyl betaine may be due to amidoamine: a patch test and product use test study. Contact Dermatitis. 1997;37:276–81.
111. Fowler Jr JF, Zug KM, Taylor JS, Storrs FJ, Sherertz EA, Sasseville DA, et al. Allergy to cocamidopropyl betaine and amidoamine in North America. Dermatitis. 2004;15:5–6.
112. Foti C, Bonamonte D, Mascolo G, Corcelli A, Lobasso S, Rigano L, et al. The role of 3-dimethylaminopropylamine and amidoamine in contact allergy to cocamidopropylbetaine. Contact Dermatitis. 2003;48:194–8.
113. Angelini G, Foti C, Rigano L, Vena GA. 3-Dimethylaminopropylamine: a key substance in contact allergy to cocamidopropylbetaine? Contact Dermatitis. 1995;32:96–9.
114. Hunter JE, Fowler JF. Safety to human skin of cocamidopropyl betaine: a mild surfactant for personal-care products. J Surfact Deterg. 1998;1(2):235–9.
115. Jacob SE, Chimento S. Focus on T.R.U.E. test allergen #7: colophony. Skin Aging. 2005;13(9):25–8.
116. Wöhrl S, Hemmer W, Focke M, et al. The significance of fragrance mix, balsam of Peru, colophony and propolis as screening tools in the detection of fragrance allergy. Br J Dermatol. 2001;145:268–73.

117. Rietschel R, Fowler JF. Fisher's contact dermatitis. 6th ed. Hamilton: BC Decker Inc; 2008. p. 419.
118. Jacob SE, Zapolinski T. Focus on: compositae. Skin Aging. 2007;15(6):44–7.
119. Mittra S, Datta A, Singh K, Singh A. 5-Hydroxytyptamine-inhibiting property of feverfew: role of parthenolide content. Acta Pharmacol Sin. 2000;21(12):1106–14.
120. Paulsen E, Andersen KE, Brandao FM, Bruynzeel DP, Ducombs G, Frosch PJ, Goossens A, Lahti A, Menne T, Shaw S, Tosti A, Wahlberg JE, Wilkinson JD, Wrangsjo K. Routine patch testing with the sesquiterpene lactone mix in Europe: a 2-year experience. A multicentre study of the EECDRG. Contact Dermatitis. 1999;40(2):72–6.
121. Orion E, Paulsen E, Andersen KE, Menne T. Comparison of simultaneous patch testing with parthenolide and sesquiterpene lactone mix. Contact Dermatitis. 1998;38:207–8.
122. Lundh K, Hindsen M, Gruvberger B, Moller H, Svensson A, Bruze M. Contact allergy to herbal teas derived from Asteraceae plants. Contact Dermatitis. 2006;54(4):196–201.
123. Rodriquez-Serna M, Sanchez-Motilla JM, Ramon R, Aliaga A. Allergic and systemic contact dermatitis from *Matricaria chamomilla* tea. Contact Dermatitis. 1998;39:192–209.
124. Mahajan VK, Sharma NL, Chander Sharma R. Parthenium dermatitis: is it a systemic contact dermatitis or an airborne contact dermatitis? Contact Dermatitis. 2004;51:231–4.
125. Hausen BM, Osmundsen PE. Contact allergy to parthenolide in *Tanacetum parthenium* (L.) schulz-Bip. (Feverfew, *Asteraceae*) and cross-reactions to related sesquiterpene lactone containing *Compositae* species. Acta Derm Venereol. 1983;63(4):308–14.
126. Paulsen E, Andersen KE, Hausen BM. Sensitization and cross-reaction patterns in Danish Compositae-allergic patients. Contact Dermatitis. 2001;45(4):197–204.
127. Davis MD, El-Azhary RA, Farmer SA. Results of patch testing to a corticosteroid series: a retrospective review of 1188 patients during 6 years at Mayo Clinic. J Am Acad Dermatol. 2007;56:921–7.
128. Coopman S, et al. Identification of cross-reaction patterns in allergic contact dermatitis from topical corticosteroids. Br J Dermatol. 1989;121:27–34.
129. Rycroft RJE et al., eds. Textbook of contact dermatitis. 3rd ed. Berlin: Springer; 2001.
130. Jacob SE, Steele T. Corticosteroid classes: a quick reference guide including patch test substances and cross reactivity. J Am Acad Dermatol. 2006;54(4):723–7.
131. Jacob SE, Steele T. Focus on allergen of the year 2005: corticosteroids. Skin Aging. 2006;33–6.
132. Baeck M, Goossens A. New insights about delayed allergic hypersensitivity to corticosteroids. G Ital Dermatol Venereol. 2012;147(1):65–9.

133. Cohen DE, Brancaccio R. What is new in clinical research in contact dermatitis. Dermatol Clin. 1997;15:137–48.
134. Boffa MJ, Wilkinson SM, Beck HM. Screening for corticosteroid contact hypersensitivity. Contact Dermatitis. 1995;33:149–51.
135. Coopman S, Degreef H, Dooms-Goossens A. Identification of cross-reaction patterns in allergic contact dermatitis from topical corticosteroids. Br J Dermatol. 1989;121:27–34.
136. Wilkinson SM. Corticosteroid cross-reactions: an alternative view. Contact Dermatitis. 2000;42:59–63.
137. Foti C, Bonifazi E, Casulli C, Bonamonte D, Conserva A, Angelini G. Contact allergy to topical corticosteroids in children with atopic dermatitis. Contact Dermatitis. 2005;52:162–3.
138. Jacob SE, Brod B, Crawford GH. Clinically relevant patch test reactions in children – a United States based study. Pediatr Dermatol. 2008;25(5):520–7.
139. Mimesh S, Pratt M. Allergic contact dermatitis from corticosteroids: reproducibility of patch testing and correlation with intradermal testing. Dermatitis. 2006;17:137–42.
140. Isaksson M, Bruze M, Lepoittevin JP, Goossens A. Patch testing with serial dilutions of budesonide, its R and S diastereomers, and potentially cross-reacting substances. Am J Contact Dermat. 2001;12:170–6.
141. Bruze M, Zimerson E. Dimethyl fumarate. Dermatitis. 2011;22(1):3–7.
142. Giménez-Arnau A. Dimethyl fumarate: a human health hazard. Dermatitis. 2011;22(1):47–9.
143. Stefanelli P, Barbini DA, Girolimetti S, Santilio A, Dommarco R. Determination of dimethyl fumarate (DMFu) in silica gel pouches using gas chromatography coupled ion trap mass spectrometry. J Environ Sci Health B. 2011;46(4):341–9.
144. Gennari O, Montesano D, Salzano A, Albrizio S, Grumetto L. Determination of dimethyl fumarate in desiccant and antimould sachets by reversed-phase liquid chromatography. Biomed Chromatogr. 2011;25(12):1315–8.
145. D'Erme AM, Bassi A, Lotti T, Gola M. Dimethyl fumarate contact dermatitis of the foot: an increasingly widespread disease. Int J Dermatol. 2012;51(1):42–5. doi:10.1111/j.1365-4632.2011.04916.x.
146. Lo Balbo A, Gotelli MJ, Mac Cormack WP, Kogan N, Gotelli C. Contact dermatitis caused by dimethylfumarate in Argentina. Clin Toxicol (Phila). 2011;49(6):508–9.
147. Silvestre JF, Toledo F, Mercader P, Giménez-Arnau AM. A summary of shoe allergic contact dermatitis caused by dimethyl fumarate in Spain. Contact Dermatitis. 2011;65(2):122–3.
148. Commission decision of 17 March 2009 requiring member states to ensure that products containing the biocide dimethyl fumarate are not placed or made available on the market. Off J Eur Union. 2009;52:32–4.

149. Lazarov A, Trattner A, David M, Ingber A. Textile dermatitis in Israel: a retrospective study. Am J Contact Dermat. 2000;11:26–9.
150. Pratt M, Taraska V. Disperse blue dyes 106 and 124 are common causes of textile dermatitis and should serve as screening allergens for this condition. Am J Contact Dermat. 2000;11:30–41.
151. Giusti F, Massone F, Bertoni L, Pellacani G, Seidenari S. Contact sensitization to disperse dyes in children. Pediatr Dermatol. 2003;20:393–7.
152. Alberta L, Sweeney SM, Wiss K. Diaper dye dermatitis. Pediatrics. 2005;116:e450–2.
153. Batchelor RJ, Wilkinson SM. Contact allergy to disperse dyes in plastic spectacle frames. Contact Dermatitis. 2006;54:66–7.
154. Guin JD. Seat-belt dermatitis from disperse blue dyes. Contact Dermatitis. 2001;44:263.
155. Jacob SE, Steele T. Focus on T.R.U.E. test allergen #14: epoxy. Skin Aging. 2006;18–20, 22.
156. Summerfield W, Goodson A, Cooper I. Survey of bisphenol a diglycidyl ether (BADGE) in canned foods. Food Addit Contam. 1998;15(7):818–30.
157. Jacob SE, Ballard CJ. Focus on T.R.U.E. test allergen #11: ethylenediamine. Skin Aging. 2006;19–22.
158. Lands AM, Hoppe JO. The toxicologic properties of N,N-dimethyl-N'-(3-thenyl)-N'-(2-pyridyl)ethylenediamine hydrochloride (thenfadil) a new antihistaminic drug. J Pharmacol Exp Ther. 1949;97(3):371–8.
159. Scheman AJ, Carroll PA, Brown KH, Osburn AH. Formaldehyde-related textile allergy: an update. Contact Dermatitis. 1998;38:332–6.
160. Rietschel RL. Experience with supplemental allergens in the diagnosis of contact dermatitis. Contact Dermatitis. 2000;65:27–30.
161. Fowler Jr JF, Skinner SM, Belsito DV. Allergic contact dermatitis from formaldehyde resins in permanent press clothing: an underdiagnosed cause of generalized dermatitis. J Am Acad Dermatol. 1992;27:962–8.
162. DeGroot AC, Maibach HI. Does allergic contact dermatitis from formaldehyde in clothes treated with durable-press chemical finishes exist in the USA? Contact Dermatitis. 2010;62:127–36.
163. Trattner A, Johansen JD, Menné T. Formaldehyde concentration in diagnostic patch testing: comparison of 1 % with 2 %. Contact Dermatitis. 1998;38:9–13.
164. Jacob SE, Steele T, Rodriguez G. Focus on T.R.U.E. test allergens # 21, 13, and 18: formaldehyde, p-tert butylphenol formaldehyde resin and quaternium 15. Skin Aging. 2005; 22–5.
165. Moennich JN, Hanna DM, Jacob SE. Formaldehyde-releasing preservative in baby and cosmetic products: health risks related to exposure during infancy. J Dermatol Nurs. 2009;1(3):211–4.
166. Jacob SE, Steele T. Avoiding formaldehyde allergic reactions in children. Pediatr Ann. 2007;36(1):55–6.

167. Jordan Jr WP, Sherman WT, King SE. Threshold responses in formaldehyde-sensitive subjects. J Am Acad Dermatol. 1979;1: 44–8.
168. Russell K, Jacob SE. Sodium hydroxymethylglycinate. Dermatitis. 2010;21(2):109–10.
169. Scientific Committee on Cosmetic Products and Non-Food Products Intended for Consumers. Opinion concerning a clarification on the formaldehyde and para-formaldehyde entry in directive 76/768/EEC on cosmetic products. SCCNFP/587/02, final. Adopted by the SCCNFP during the 22nd plenary meeting of 17 December 2002. http://ec.europa.eu/health/ph_risk/committees/sccp/documents/out187_en.pdf. Accessed 22 Mar 2011.
170. De Groot AC, White IR, Flyvholm M, Lensen G, Coenraads P. Formaldehyde-releasers in cosmetics: relationship to formaldehyde contact allergy: part 1. Characterization, frequency and relevance of sensitization, and frequency of use in cosmetics. Contact Dermatitis. 2010;62:2–17.
171. Herbert C, Rietschel RL. Formaldehyde and formaldehyde releasers: How much avoidance of cross-reacting agents is required? Contact Dermatitis. 2004;50(6):371–3.
172. Habeck M. Formaldehyde. 2010. [1 screen]. Eco-USA.net. http://www.ecousa.net/toxics/chemicals/formaldehyde.shtml. Accessed 22 Mar 2011.
173. Maier LE, Lampel HP, Bhutani T, Jacob SE. Hand dermatitis: a focus on allergic contact dermatitis to biocides. Dermatol Clin. 2009;27(3):251–64, v–vi.
174. Cook P, Sleeker C. Bakelite: an illustrated guide to collectible bakelite objects. Secaucus/ New York: Chartwell Books; 1992.
175. Restani P, Campagner P, Fiecchi A, et al. Identification of spinacine as the principal reaction product of gamma-casein with formaldehyde in cheese. Food Chem Toxicol. 1988;26(5):441–6.
176. Hill AM, Belsito DV. Systemic contact dermatitis of the eyelids caused by formaldehyde derived from aspartame. Contact Dermatitis. 2003;49(5):258–9.
177. Poliovirus Vaccine Inactivated IPOL. U.S. food and drug administration. 2005. 1 screen. http://www.fda.gov/downloads/Biologics-BloodVaccines/Vaccines/ApprovedProducts/UCM133479.pdf. Accessed 22 Mar 2011.
178. BioThrax® (Anthrax Vaccine Adsorbed). U.S. food and drug administration. 16 screens. http://www.fda.gov/downloads/Biologics-BloodVaccines/BloodBloodProducts/ApprovedProducts/LicensedProductsBLAs/UCM074923.pdf. Accessed 22 Mar 2011.
179. Diphtheria and Tetanus Toxoids and Acellular Pertussis Vaccine Adsorbed Tripedia®. U.S. food and drug administration. 2005. 13 screens. http://www.fda.gov/downloads/Biologics-BloodVaccines/Vaccines/ApprovedProducts/UCM101580.pdf. Accessed 22 Mar 2011.

180. Havrix (Hepatitis A Vaccine). U.S. food and drug administration. 2010. 15 screens. http://www.fda.gov/downloads/BiologicsBlood Vaccines/Vaccines/ApprovedProducts/UCM224555.pdf. Accessed 22 Mar 2011.
181. Zug KA, Warshaw EM, Fowler JF, et al. Patch-test results of the North American Contact Dermatitis Group 2005–2006. Dermatitis. 2009;20(3):149–60.
182. Herro EM, Elsaie ML, Nijhawan RI, Jacob SE. Comparison of allergens in allergic contact eyelid dermatitis – recommendations for a screening series. Dermatitis. 2012;23(1):17–20.
183. Jacob SE, Maldonado EA, Herro EM. Allergen focus: formaldehyde and formaldehyde releasing preservatives revisited. Skin Aging. 2011;19(6):24–7.
184. Bardana Jr EJ, Montanaro A. Formaldehyde: an analysis of its respiratory, cutaneous, and immunologic effects. Ann Allergy. 1991;66(6):441–52.
185. Agner T, Flyvholm MA, Menne T. Formaldehyde allergy: a follow-up study. Am J Contact Dermat. 1999;10:12–7.
186. Trocho C, Pardo R, Rafecas I, et al. Formaldehyde derived from dietary aspartame binds to tissue components in vivo. Life Sci. 1998;63(5):337–49.
187. Jacob SE, Stechschulte S. Formaldehyde, aspartame and migraines: a possible connection. Dermatitis. 2008;19(3):E10–1.
188. Fransway AF, Schmitz NA. The problem of preservation in the 1990s. II. Formaldehyde and formaldehyde releasing biocides: incidences of cross-reactivity and the significance of the positive response to formaldehyde. Am J Contact Dermat. 1991;2:78–88.
189. Baker RR. The generation of formaldehyde in cigarettes: overview and recent experiments. Food Chem Toxicol. 2006;44(11):1799–822.
190. Andersen K, White I, Goossens A. Allergens from the standard series. In: Rycroft R, Menne T, Frosch P, Lepoittevin JP, editors. Textbook of contact dermatitis. 3rd ed. New York: Springer; 2001.
191. Sasseville D. Hypersensitivity to preservatives. Dermatol Ther. 2004;17(3):251–63.
192. Jacob SE, Hsu JW. Sodium hydroxymethylglycinate: a potential formaldehyde-releasing preservative in child products. Dermatitis. 2009;10(6):347–9.
193. Rietschel R, Fowler JF. Fisher's contact dermatitis. 6th ed. Hamilton: BC Decker Inc; 2008. p. 268–9.
194. Warshaw EM, Ahmed RL, Belsito DV, et al. Contact dermatitis of the hands: cross-sectional analyses of North American contact dermatitis group data, 1994–2004. J Am Acad Dermatol. 2007;57:301–14.
195. Jacob SE, Amado A. Focus on T.R.U.E. test allergen #6: fragrance mix. Skin Aging. 2006;14(4):16–8, 22.

References

196. Chatard H. Case of sensitization to perfumes with cutaneous and general reactions. Bull Soc Fr Dermatol Syphiligr. 1957;64(3):323.
197. Larsen WG. Perfume dermatitis. A study of 20 patients. Arch Dermatol. 1977;113(5):623–6.
198. Johansen JD. Fragrance contact allergy: a clinical review. Am J Clin Dermatol. 2003;4(11):789–98.
199. Militello G, James W. Lyral: a fragrance allergen. Dermatitis. 2005;16(1):41–4.
200. Scheinman PL. The foul side of fragrance-free products: what every clinician should know about managing patients with fragrance allergy. J Am Acad Dermatol. 1999;41(6):1020–4.
201. Food and Drugs. Food and Drug Administration Department of Health and Human Services. Code of Federal Regulations. http://www.accessdata.fda.gov/scripts/cdrh/cfdocs/cfcfr/CFRSearch.cfm?CFRPart=700&showFR=1. Accessed 25 Jan 2006.
202. Jacob SE, Amado A. Focus on T.R.U.E. test allergen #10: balsam of Peru. Skin Aging. 2005;13(3):23–4.
203. Smith WJ, Jacob SE. The role of allergic contact dermatitis in diaper dermatitis. Pediatr Dermatol. 2009;26(3):369–70.
204. Patch Test Products 2011. Chemotechnique diagnostics. 2011. http://www.chemotechnique.se/Catalogue.htm. Accessed 28 Mar 2011.
205. Rietschel R, Fowler JF. Fisher's contact dermatitis. 6th ed. Hamilton: BC Decker Inc; 2008. p. 552.
206. Warshaw EM, Schram SE, Maibach HI, Belsito DV, Marks Jr JG, Fowler Jr JF, Rietschel RL, Taylor JS, Mathias CG, DeLeo VA, Zug KA, Sasseville D, Storrs FJ, Pratt MD. Occupation-related contact dermatitis in North American health care workers referred for patch testing: cross-sectional data, 1998 to 2004. Dermatitis. 2008;19(5):261–74.
207. Shaffer MP, Belsito DV. Allergic contact dermatitis from glutaraldehyde in health-care workers. Contact Dermatitis. 2000;43(3):150–6. Review.
208. Ravis SM, Shaffer MP, Shaffer CL, Dehkhaghani S, Belsito DV. Glutaraldehyde-induced and formaldehyde-induced allergic contact dermatitis among dental hygienists and assistants. J Am Dent Assoc. 2003;134(8):1072–8.
209. Marks JG, DeLeo VA, editors. Contact and occupational dermatology. 2nd ed. St Louis: Mosby; 1997.
210. Rietschel RL, Warshaw EM, Sasseville D, Fowler JF, DeLeo VA, Belsito DV, Taylor JS, Storrs FJ, Mathias CG, Maibach HI, Marks JG, Zug KA, Pratt M, North American Contact Dermatitis Group. Common contact allergens associated with eyelid dermatitis: data from the North American Contact Dermatitis Group 2003–2004 study period. Dermatitis. 2007;18(2):78–81.
211. Laeijendecker R, van Joost T. Oral manifestations of gold allergy. J Am Acad Dermatol. 1994;30(2 Pt 1):205–9.

212. Nedorost S, Wagman A. Positive patch-test reactions to gold: patients' perception of relevance and the role of titanium dioxide in cosmetics. Dermatitis. 2005;16(2):67–70.
213. Jacob SE, Rouhani P. Focus on allergen of the year 2001: gold. Skin Aging. 2006;16–22.
214. Henriks-Eckerman ML, Suuronen K, Jolanki R. Analysis of allergens in metalworking fluids. Contact Dermatitis. 2008;59(5):261–7.
215. Warshaw EM, Belsito DV, DeLeo VA, Fowler Jr JF, Maibach HI, Marks JG, Toby Mathias CG, Pratt MD, Rietschel RL, Sasseville D, Storrs FJ, Taylor JS, Zug KA. North American Contact Dermatitis Group patch-test results, 2003–2004 study period. Dermatitis. 2008;19(3):129–36.
216. Bryld LE, Agner T, Menné T. Allergic contact dermatitis from 3-iodo-2-propynyl-butylcarbamate (IPBC) – an update. Contact Dermatitis. 2001;44(5):276–8.
217. Schnuch A, Geier J, Brasch J, Uter W. The preservative iodopropynyl butylcarbamate: frequency of allergic reactions and diagnostic considerations. Contact Dermatitis. 2002;46(3):153–6.
218. Brasch J, Schnuch A, Geier J, Aberer W, Uter W, German Contact Dermatitis Research Group, Information Network of Departments of Dermatology. Iodopropynylbutyl carbamate 0.2 % is suggested for patch testing of patients with eczema possibly related to preservatives. Br J Dermatol. 2004;151(3):608–15.
219. Lanigan RS. Final report on the safety assessment of iodopropynyl butylcarbamate (IPBC). Int J Toxicol. 1998;17(5):1–37.
220. Hasan T, Rantanen T, Alanko K, Harvima RJ, Jolanki R, Kalimo K, et al. Patch test reactions to cosmetic allergens in 1995–1997 and 2000–2002 in Finland–a multicentre study. Contact Dermatitis. 2005;53:40–5.
221. Wakelin SH, Smith H, White IR, Rycroft RJ, McFadden JP. A retrospective analysis of contact allergy to lanolin. Br J Dermatol. 2001;145:28–31.
222. Jacob SE, Ai J. Focus on T.R.U.E. test allergen #2: lanolin-wool wax. Skin Aging. 2005;13(1):25–6.
223. Castanedo-Tardan MP, Jacob SE. Allergic contact dermatitis to sorbitan sesquioleate in children. Contact Dermatitis. 2008;58(3):171–2.
224. Pratt MD, Belsito DV, DeLeo VA, Fowler Jr JF, Fransway AF, Maibach HI, et al. North American Contact Dermatitis Group patch-test results, 2001–2002 study period. Dermatitis. 2004;15(1):25–32.
225. Marks J, et al. MCI/MI (Kathon CG) biocide – United States multicenter study of human skin sensitization. Am J Contact Dermat. 1990;1:157.

226. De Groot AC, Weyland JW. Contact allergy to MDGN in the cosmetics preservative Euxyl K400. Am J Contact Dermat. 1991;2:31–2.
227. Schnuch A, Geier J, Uter W, Frosch PJ. Patch testing with preservatives, antimicrobials and industrial biocides. Results from a multicentre study. Br J Dermatol. 1998;138(3):467–76.
228. Nguyen SH, Dang TP, MacPherson C, Maibach HI. Prevalence of patch test results from 1970 to 2002 in a multi-centre population in North America. Contact Dermatitis. 2008;58:101–6.
229. Chambers HF. Aminoglycosides & spectinomycin. In: Katzung BG, editor. Basic and clinical pharmacology. 9th ed. New York: Lange Medical/McGraw-Hill; 2004.
230. Jacob SE, Herrick D. Focus on T.R.U.E. test allergen #3:neomycin. Skin Aging. 2005;13(8):26–8.
231. Spann CT, Tutrone WD, Weinberg JM, Scheinfeld N, Ross B. Topical antibacterial agents for wound care: a primer. Dermatol Surg. 2003;29(6):620–6.
232. Leventhal JS, Berger EM, Brauer JA, Cohen DE. Hypersensitivity reactions to vaccine constituents: a case series and review of the literature. Dermatitis. 2012;23(3):102–9. doi:10.1097/DER.0b013e31825228cf.
233. Jacob SE, James WD. From road rash to top allergen in a flash: bacitracin. Dermatol Surg. 2004;30:521–4.
234. Agathos M. Anaphylactic reaction to framycetin (neomycin B) and lignocaine. Contact Dermatitis. 1980;6(3):236–7.
235. Veien NK. Ingested food in systemic allergic contact dermatitis. Clin Dermatol. 1997;15:547–55.
236. de Menezes Padua CA, Schnuch A, Lessmann H, Geier J, Pfahlberg A, Uter W. Contact allergy to neomycin sulfate: results of a multifactorial analysis. Pharmacoepidemiol Drug Saf. 2005;14(10):725–33.
237. Barceloux DG. Nickel. J Toxicol Clin Toxicol. 1999;37(2):239–58. Erratum in: J Toxicol Clin Toxicol 2000;38(7):813.
238. Pratt MD, Belsito DV, DeLeo VA, Fowler Jr JF, Fransway AF, Maibach HI, et al. North American Contact Dermatitis Group patch-test results, 2001–2002 study period. Dermatitis. 2004;15:176–83.
239. Jacob SE, Amado A. Focus on T.R.U.E. test allergen #1: nickel. Skin Aging. 2005;13(5):21–4.
240. Herro EM, Russell K, Jacob SE. The common presentations of allergic contact dermatitis in children: a guide to diagnosis and management. Pract Dermatol Pediatr. 2010;27–34.
241. Wöhrl S, Jandl T, Stingl G, Kinaciyan T. Mobile telephone as new source for nickel dermatitis. Contact Dermatitis. 2007;56:113.
242. Livideanu C, Giordano-Labadie F, Paul C. Cellular phone addiction and allergic contact dermatitis to nickel. Contact Dermatitis. 2007;57:130–1.

243. Veien NK, Hattel T, Laurberg G. Low nickel diet: an open, prospective trial. J Am Acad Dermatol. 1993;29(6):1002–7.
244. Arnich N, Sirot V, Riviere G, Jean J, Noel L, Guerin T, Leblanc JC. Dietary exposure to trace elements and health risk assessment in the 2nd French Total Diet Study. Food Chem Toxicol. 2012;50(7):2432–49.
245. Rietschel R, Fowler JF. Fisher's contact dermatitis. 6th ed. Hamilton: BC Decker Inc; 2008. p. 672.
246. Dotterud LK, Falk ES. Metal allergy in north Norwegian schoolchildren and its relationship with ear piercing and atopy. Contact Dermatitis. 1994;31:308–13.
247. Nakamura M, Arima Y, Nobuhara S, Miyachi Y. Nickel allergy in a trumpet player. Contact Dermatitis. 1999;40:219–20.
248. Moennich JN, Zirwas M, Jacob SE. Nickel-induced facial dermatitis: adolescents beware of the cell phone. Cutis. 2009;84(4):199–200.
249. Silvestri DL, Barmettler S. Pruritus ani as a manifestation of systemic contact dermatitis: resolution with dietary nickel restriction. Dermatitis. 2011;22(1):50–5.
250. Hsu JW, Jacob SE. Children's toys as potential sources of nickel exposure. Dermatitis. 2009;20(6):349–50.
251. Veien NK. Systemic contact dermatitis. Int J Dermatol. 2011;50(12):1445–56.
252. Guy et al. Metals and the skin, topical effects and systemic absorption. New York: Marcel Dekker; 1999. p. 307.
253. Neri I, Guareschi E, Savoia F, Patrizi A. Childhood allergic contact dermatitis from henna tattoo. Pediatr Dermatol. 2002;19(6):503–5.
254. Chung WH, Chang YC, Yang LJ, Hung SI, Lin JY, et al. Clinicopathologic features of skin reactions to temporary tattoos and analysis of possible causes. Arch Dermatol. 2002;138(1):88–92.
255. Brancaccio RR, Brown LH, Chang YT, Fogelman JP, Mafong EA, Cohen DE. Identification and quantification of para-phenylenediamine in a temporary black henna tattoo. Am J Contact Dermat. 2002;13:15–8.
256. Sosted H, Johansen JD, Andersen KE, et al. Severe allergic hair dye reactions in 8 children. Contact Dermatitis. 2006;54:87–91.
257. Jacob SE, Zapolanski T, Chayavichitsilp P, Connelly EA, Eichenfield LF. p-Phenylenediamine in black henna tattoos: a practice in need of policy in children. Arch Pediatr Adolesc Med. 2008;162(8):790–2.
258. Leysat SD, Boone M, Blondeel A, Song M. Two cases of cross-sensitivity in subjects allergic to paraphenylenediamine following ingestion of polaronil. Dermatology. 2003;206:379–80.
259. Arroyo MP. Black henna tattoo reaction in a person with sulfonamide and benzocaine allergy. J Am Acad Dermatol. 2003;48(2):301–2.

260. Geldof BA, Roesyanto ID, van Joost TH. Clinical aspects of para-tertiary-butylphenolformaldehyde resin. Contact Dermatitis. 1989;21:312–5.
261. Herro EM, Friedlander SF, Jacob SE. Bra associated allergic contact dermatitis: p-tert-butylphenol formaldehyde resin as the culprit. Pediatr Dermatol. 2012;29(4):540–1.
262. Rietschel R, Fowler JF. Fisher's contact dermatitis. 6th ed. Hamilton: BC Decker Inc; 2008. p. 274–5.
263. Biebl KA, Warshaw EM. Allergic contact dermatitis to cosmetics. Dermatol Clin. 2006;24(2):215–32, vii.
264. Cashman AL, Warshaw EM. Parabens: a review of epidemiology, structure, allergenicity, and hormonal properties. Dermatitis. 2005;16(2):57–66; quiz 55–6.
265. Castanedo-Tardan MP, Jacob SE. Potassium dichromate. Dermatitis. 2008;19(4):E24–5.
266. Jacob SE, Amado A. Focus on T.R.U.E. test allergen #4:chromates. Skin Aging. 2005;13(11):21–3.
267. Veien NK, Hattel T, Justesen O, Norholm A. Oral challenge with metal salts. (I). Vesicular patch-test-negative hand eczema. Contact Dermatitis. 1983;9:402–6.
268. Holden CR, Gawkrodger DJ. 10 years' experience of patch testing with a shoe series in 230 patients: which allergens are important? Contact Dermatitis. 2005;53:37–9.
269. Warshaw EM, Schram SE, Belsito DV, DeLeo VA, Fowler Jr JF, Maibach HI, et al. Shoe allergens: retrospective analysis of cross-sectional data from the North American contact dermatitis group, 2001–2004. Dermatitis. 2007;18:191–202.
270. Lowther A, McCormick T, Nedorost S. Systemic contact dermatitis from propylene glycol. Dermatitis. 2008;19(2):105–8.
271. Ownby DR. A history of latex allergy. J Allergy Clin Immunol. 2002;110:s27–32.
272. Hosler D, Burkett SL, Tarkanian MJ. Prehistoric polymers: rubber processing in ancient Mesoamerica. Science. 1999;284:1988–91.
273. Slack C. Noble obsession: Charles Goodyear, Thomas Hancock, and the race to unlock the greatest industrial secret of the nineteenth century. New York: Hyperion; 2003.
274. Jacob SE, Villafradez-Diaz LM. Focus on T.R.U.E. test allergen #15: carbamates. Skin Aging. 2005;13(10):26–30.
275. Cronin E. Shoe dermatitis. Br J Dermatol. 1966;78(12):617–25.
276. Marks J, DeLeo V. Standard allergens. In: Contact and occupational dermatology. 2nd ed. St. Louis: Mosby; 1997. p. 98–102.
277. Jacob SE, Nelson C. Focus on T.R.U.E. test allergen #19 & #22: mercaptobenzothiazole and mercapto mix. Skin Aging. 2006;14(9):19–20, 22, 24, 26.

278. Jacob SE, Dimson O. Focus on T.R.U.E. test allergen #24: thiuram. Skin Aging. 2006;14(2):44, 49–50.
279. Jacob SE, Anderson. Focus on NACDG allergen: mixed dialkyl thioureas. Skin Aging. 2007;15:16–8.
280. Roul S, Ducombs G, Leaute-Labreze C, Taieb A. "Lucky Luke" contact dermatitis due to rubber components of diapers. Contact Dermatitis. 1998;38(6):363–4.
281. Belhadjali H, Giordano-Labadie F, Rance F, Bazex J. "Lucky Luke" contact dermatitis from diapers: a new allergen? Contact Dermatitis. 2001;44(4):248.
282. Jordan WP, Bourlas MC. Allergic contact dermatitis to underwear elastic. Chemically transformed by laundry bleach. Arch Dermatol. 1975;111:593–5.
283. Martensen-Larsen O. Five years' experience with disulfiram in the treatment of alcoholics. Q J Stud Alcohol. 1953;14(3):406–18.
284. Fisher AA. Allergic reactions to nonrubber products by testing with rubber mixes. Part II: the mercapto mix. Cutis. 1995;56:197.
285. Bonnevie P, Marcussen P. Rubber products as a widespread cause of eczema. Report of 80 cases. Acta Derm Venereol. 1944;25:163–78.
286. Castanedo-Tardan MP, Jacob SE. Sorbitan sesquioleate. Dermatitis. 2008;19(4):E22–3.
287. Asarch A, Scheinman PL. Sorbitan sesquioleate, a common emulsifier in topical corticosteroids, is an important contact allergen. Dermatitis. 2008;19(6):323–7.
288. Jacob SE, Huo R. Focus on T.R.U.E. test allergen #23: thimerosal. Skin Aging. 2006;14:16–18, 21.
289. Engler DE. Mercury "bleaching" creams. J Am Acad Dermatol. 2005;52(6):1113–4.
290. Breithaupt A, Jacob SE. Thimerosal and the relevance of patch-test reactions in children. Dermatitis. 2008;19(5):275–7.
291. Tsuruta D, Sowa J, Higashi N, Kobayashi H, Ishii M. A red tattoo and a swordfish supper. Lancet. 2004;364(9435):730.
292. Fisher AA. Contact dermatitis. 3rd ed. Philadelphia: Lea & Febiger; 1986. p. 383–4.
293. Elder RL. Final report on the safety assessment of toluenesulfonamide/formaldehyde resin. Int J Toxicol. 1986;5(5):471–90.
294. Stechschulte SA, Avashia N, Jacob SE. Tosylamide formaldehyde resin. Dermatitis. 2008;19(3):E18–9.